#24
Canoga Park Branch Library
20939 Sherman Way
Canoga Park, CA 91303

The
Stroke
Book

ALSO BY JUNE BIERMANN AND BARBARA TOOHEY

The Diabetic's Total Health and Happiness Book

The Woman's Holistic Headache Relief Book

The Diabetic's Sports and Exercise Book

The Diabetic's Book: All Your Questions Answered

The Peripatetic Diabetic

The Diabetic Woman
(with Lois Jovanovic, M.D.)

The Diabetic Man
(with Peter Lodewick, M.D.)

Psyching Out Diabetes
(with Richard R. Rubin, Ph.D.)

Diabetes Type 2 and What to Do
(with Virginia Valentine, R.N., MSN, CDE)

UNDER THE NAME MARGARET BENNETT

Biking for Grown-ups

Cross-Country Skiing for the Fun of It

How to Ski Just a Little Bit

Dr. Owl's Problem

From Baedeker to Worse

Alice in Womanland

TWENTY-FOUR   JUL 1 1 2005

The Stroke Book

A GUIDE TO LIFE AFTER STROKE
FOR SURVIVORS AND THOSE
WHO CARE FOR THEM

**June Biermann
and Barbara Toohey**

616.81
B588

Jeremy P. Tarcher/Penguin
a member of Penguin Group (USA) Inc.
New York

1611 1274 4

JEREMY P. TARCHER/PENGUIN
Published by the Penguin Group
Penguin Group (USA) Inc., 375 Hudson Street, New York, New York 10014, USA ·
Penguin Group (Canada), 10 Alcorn Avenue, Toronto, Ontario M4V 3B2, Canada (a division
of Pearson Penguin Canada Inc.) · Penguin Books Ltd, 80 Strand, London WC2R 0RL,
England · Penguin Ireland, 25 St Stephen's Green, Dublin 2, Ireland (a division of Penguin
Books Ltd) · Penguin Group (Australia), 250 Camberwell Road, Camberwell, Victoria 3124,
Australia (a division of Pearson Australia Group Pty Ltd) · Penguin Books India Pvt Ltd,
11 Community Centre, Panchsheel Park, New Delhi–110 017, India · Penguin Group (NZ),
Cnr Airborne and Rosedale Roads, Albany, Auckland 1310, New Zealand (a division of Pearson
New Zealand Ltd) · Penguin Books (South Africa) (Pty) Ltd, 24 Sturdee Avenue, Rosebank,
Johannesburg 2196, South Africa · Penguin Books Ltd, Registered Offices:
80 Strand, London WC2R 0RL, England

Copyright © 2005 by June Biermann and Barbara Toohey
All rights reserved. No part of this book may be reproduced, scanned, or distributed in any printed
or electronic form without permission. Please do not participate in or encourage piracy of
copyrighted materials in violation of the author's rights. Purchase only authorized editions.
Published simultaneously in Canada

Most Tarcher/Penguin books are available at special quantity discounts for bulk purchase for sales pro-
motions, premiums, fund-raising, and educational needs. Special books or book excerpts also can be
created to fit specific needs. For details, write Penguin Group (USA) Inc. Special Markets, 375 Hudson
Street, New York, NY 10014.

Library of Congress Cataloging-in-Publication Data

Biermann, June.
    The stroke book: a guide to life after stroke for survivors and those who care for them /
June Biermann and Barbara Toohey.
       p.   cm.
    Includes index.
    ISBN 1-58542-374-2
    1. Cerebrovascular disease—Popular works. I. Toohey, Barbara. II. Title.

RC388.5.B54   2004   2004058020
616.8'103—dc22

Printed in the United States of America

10   9   8   7   6   5   4   3   2

This book is printed on acid-free paper. ♾

Book design by Tanya Maiboroda

Neither the publisher nor the author is engaged in rendering professional advice or services to the individual reader. The ideas, procedures, and suggestions contained in this book are not intended as a substitute
for consulting with your physician. All matters regarding your health require medical supervision. Neither the author nor the publisher shall be liable or responsible for any loss or damage allegedly arising
from any information or suggestion in this book.

While the author has made every effort to provide accurate telephone numbers and Internet addresses
at the time of publication, neither the publisher nor the author assumes any responsibility for errors, or
for changes that occur after publication.

To June, who, with her manifold health problems, keeps
giving us ideas and material for our books. But enough is enough!
—*Barbara*

To Barbara for helping me live through and with
all my ailments despite my sometime efforts to thwart her.
—*June*

To Deding, skilled nurse, loving friend, and our proverbial
"beacon of light in a world of darkness." Long may she shine!
—*June and Barbara*

Contents

Acknowledgments

. . . .

We would like to express our appreciation to the following for making this book possible:

The dedicated therapists and staff members of Valley Presbyterian Hospital, Encino-Tarzana Medical Center, and Sherman Oaks Health and Rehabilitation Center. Thanks for continually gluing June back together.

Ashley Shelby, who was as much a collaborator as an editor—and a star in both roles.

Jeremy Tarcher, our longtime publisher and friend. We hope we continue doing books together throughout the millennium and into our next lives.

Foreword

. . . .

One of the great advantages of books on technical subjects written by laymen is the ability to communicate with other laymen without having to penetrate the jargon-filled arcane descriptions written by experts. This is especially true with medical issues where the author is often the one experiencing the subject at hand. Here we have a book on stroke by two women already known for producing similar works on diabetes. Barbara Toohey and June Biermann have now presented the reader with the unusual perspective of the individual who has suffered the consequence of cerebral vascular disease, as well as that of her companion. The patient's angle differs greatly from the doctor's. The doctor is concerned with diagnosis and treatment, with what tests to do and ultimately with the prognosis. The patient and caregiver are more concerned about getting along day to day, and are involved with solving the minutiae of activities of daily living. In this book you will see much more of the latter and parts that could not have been written by a doctor. The medical aspects and descriptions are of interest because they define the patient's understanding of the disease, rather than necessarily providing a distinct detailed account of the pathophysiology involved.

Much practical information is here, and this book can function as a handbook describing June's experience. The references are to local facilities but the action is universal. The fundamental consequence of a stroke is independent of location and the methods of dealing with it are similar. This is a real strength and allows the reader to adapt fundamental strategies to his own location. June and Barbara can translate directly to someone with a stroke living halfway across the world.

A stroke can be defined as the sudden onset of a focal neurological deficit. This book deals with the most common forms and will strike a chord of familiarity with most readers. By eliminating the smokescreen of the medical textbook this book can be put to good use by those without a technical background. June and Barbara's longtime experience in dealing with diabetes has made them ideal candidates for introducing this subject, for many of the psychological and physical results are similar. In addition, diabetes is a risk factor for cerebral vascular disease, and this work can in certain ways be considered a sequel to their multiple volumes on diabetes. The physician can learn much about his patient's challenges here, and this book can serve as a source for providing better care in the future.

N. Paul Rosenthal, M.D., Ph.D.
Clinical Professor of Neurology
UCLA School of Medicine

Authors' Note

. . . .

The Stroke Book is divided into two parts. Part 1 ("The Strokee Chronicles") has been designed to aid the strokee in understanding stroke, how to prevent another one, and how to navigate
the challenges ahead in recovery. It is written from June's point
of view.

Part 2 ("A Caregiver's Compendium") is a guide for those who
care for stroke survivors, written from Barbara's point of view.
This section provides guidance, information, and solace for caregivers. However, we encourage the stroke sufferer to read the caregiver section to better understand what his or her caregiver has
been asked to undertake. Likewise, the caregiver will gain a better
perspective of and understanding for the loved one he or she cares
for after reading Part 1.

In June's four years as a strokee, she's experienced all the
ups and downs and downs and ups again of post-stroke living.
She's had ischemic strokes and hemorrhagic strokes, as well as
TIAs. She's been in and out of hospitals and rehab centers, on
and off wheelchairs and walkers and canes, and up and down
the emotional roller coaster. The scenario may be familiar to
you; and then again, maybe it isn't. Many of you may be "children
of a lesser stroke" and have only experienced a few of the strokee
vicissitudes. And yet you still must cope with whatever adver-

sities you face, along with the ever-present fear of what might come next.

With this book we hope to help you—and your caregiver—contend with the impediments, be they great or small, that your stroke has left you with and show you that you can handle them with courage and hope and even humor.

Barbara's Introduction

THE WOMAN WHO HAS EVERYTHING

. . . .

June Biermann, my friend and writing collaborator for more than forty years, could be called "the woman who has everything." In her case it is not a compliment. The everythings she has are health problems. She had pretty clear sailing until the age of forty, when she was diagnosed with type 1 diabetes. Up until that time most of our writing had been humor (*Alice in Womanland: Or the Feminine Mistake*), travel (*From Baedeker to Worse*), sports (*How to Ski Just a Little Bit, Biking for Grown-ups*) and miscellaneous magazine articles on such topics as food and dining, and other fun stuff.

With the advent of June's diabetes, it looked as if the fun might be over, what with the restrictions that diabetes would put on her life. After forlornly mulling that situation over for a while, we decided that we wouldn't let June roll over and play disabled. We set out to prove you could overcome the initial despair of diabetes and go on to live a more joyful, exciting, and healthy life than ever before. Prove it we did, and chronicled our adventures (and misadventures) in *The Peripatetic Diabetic*—a title we define as "the diabetic who gets around in every sense of the word."

When you write a book on a subject, you suddenly become an expert in the field. So building on our "expertise" we wrote seven other books on diabetes along with numerous articles. We even founded two diabetes newsletters (*The Health-O-Gram* and *The*

Diabetic Reader) and started two businesses to help people with diabetes find the supplies and books they needed (The SugarFree Centers and Prana Publications). Along the way we gave speeches and talks to various diabetes groups. Everything was hunky-dory.

Then June developed another health problem: chronic headaches. Intense and incapacitating and virtually insupportable, they pounded away in her skull one third of her waking hours and occupied all of her should-be working mind. These headaches had nothing to do with her diabetes, but it took us five years of research and experimentation and myriad fruitless doctor visits to find out what they did have to do with and how to cure them. (I won't keep you in suspense. It turned out to be TMJ [temporomandibular joint] syndrome—a misaligned jaw hinge joint.) To try to help others escape from the chronic headache jungle, we wrote *The Woman's Holistic Headache Relief Book.*

Do you see a pattern emerging here? June gets a health problem. We work out how to live with it, and then we write a book about it.

Next June experienced an acute glaucoma incident caused by a lesion (a structural change) on her iris, which was first thought to be malignant. Luckily it turned out not to be, but it *did* necessitate an iridectomy—the cutting out of a small hunk of the iris. (June no longer has to have the pupil of her left eye dilated for eye exams since the doctor can look through the hole in the iris.) Because of this experience we wrote a cautionary addendum to our *Diabetes Type 2 and What to Do* book warning of the necessity of having your eyes checked for glaucoma every year.

June had just about had it with health problems. Understandably she felt it was my turn to have the next one. But it was not to be. The worst was yet to come. On the morning of July 10, 2000, June suffered a hemorrhagic stroke, that, as Eliza Doolitle would say, almost "done her in." As she was lying unconscious in the hospital, I whispered in her ear, "If you just get through this, I promise we won't have to write a book about it."

Well, she did pull through. When our publisher, Jeremy Tarcher, called to find out how she was doing, I told him I had promised her we wouldn't have to write a book about her stroke. Jeremy replied, "*I* didn't promise her."

June's Introduction

. . . .

A stroke most dolorous

—MALLORY, *Le Morte D'Arthur*

Here I sit—in a wheelchair. I can walk across the living room to the kitchen and back with the aid of a four-pronged cane and an assist from a caregiver, chanting along the way "right, left, cane, right, left, cane." My right arm is weak and my right hand has lost its cunning. Yep, it was a stroke, one of the hemorrhagic persuasion, meaning it was caused by bleeding from a ruptured blood vessel in the brain, rather than the more common blockage caused by a blood clot.

I have hope that, if I continue to work hard on my therapies—physical (legs and trunk) and occupational (arms and hands)—I may be pretty much back to normal in six months or a year, or who knows when? The only thing that's predictable about stroke recoveries is their unpredictability.

Actually, even with my physical problems, I'm in good spirits, happy just to be alive. My doctor confessed that he didn't think I'd make it. More than a third of those with my kind of stroke die within a month, and in the first year half have succumbed. But I'm also distressed because it's almost certain that I brought it on through my own stupidity—or to be a little easier on myself, my lack of information. What was the cause of the stroke? Although

I've had diabetes for over thirty years, I've worked hard at keeping my blood sugars normal. As a result, I'm totally free from complications and have excellent cardiovascular health, including good cholesterols and triglycerides. Although diabetes is a risk factor for strokes, I'm virtually certain that diabetes can't notch its gun on this one, and because of my meticulous diabetes control, my doctors tend to agree. I've figured out that I had what you might call a stroke by constipation, with an assist from stress. Let me explain. First came the stress from the death of a very old friend, old in both the terms of her age (ninety-six) and how long I had known her (sixty years). She was my high school French teacher and became a kind of surrogate mother to me. It fell upon me to write her obituary, notify her many friends, and help with the handling of her estate, which was mainly in a complex charitable trust.

I was still under this stress and in mourning when I started experiencing major constipation. I kept thinking that this, too, shall pass (!) but it didn't. I'd had a few such experiences in the past. One even required intervention in a proctologist's office. But over the years, I got by with an occasional assist from glycerin suppositories and, in the later stages of constipation, Fleet enemas. But when I turned to my Fleets this time, the impaction was so great that neither the water nor the oil variety worked its customary magic. Finally after over an hour of intense "straining at stool," as they say in medical talk, the impaction finally broke. But that was not all that broke.

Only moments later I felt the symptoms of a stroke: a weakness on my right side (I could hardly stand) and slightly slurred speech. I called my writing collaborator, Barbara, who was in the office. She immediately took me to the hospital. By the time we got there I had to be lifted onto a wheelchair and carted to the emergency room. There they did a brain scan and discovered a bleeding area that was about the size of a quarter. The next day I was moved to the critical care unit. I thought of it as solitary confinement because it had a coded entry door that had to be opened by an attendant and only close relatives (two at a time) were allowed to visit. I had no locally available relatives, but luckily my friends were up to the challenge. I immediately acquired a sister, Barbara (she has a definite family resemblance since we get our hair done by the same hairdresser). Then came a succession of cousins, nieces, and nephews.

Barbara, who was already plotting my escape, asked one of the nurses, "How long do people in her condition usually have to stay in the hospital?"

"That depends," the nurse replied.

"Depends on what?" Barbara persisted.

"Depends on the kind of insurance they have."

I began physical and occupational therapy right away. And I did so well with those that, insurance aside, the occupational therapist figured I'd be up and out of there in about two weeks.

Friends were relieved that I was coming around so quickly, and so was I. But the following day something happened, something that I can only report through the observation of others.

Suddenly I couldn't speak. I could only manage a "ruhr, ruhr, ruhr" sound, couldn't chew (food all wound up in a pocket of my cheek), couldn't swallow, couldn't move my right hand, arm, or leg. I couldn't recognize even my closest friends, and the only way people could tell that I was responding was when I was told to stick out my tongue; it would make a tentative foray between my dry lips. The hospital staff raced me down for another brain scan since they thought the blood vessel in the brain must be bleeding again. But when the scans came back it was the same old 25¢ piece. No one—not even the doctors—seemed to know the cause of this sudden downturn. One theory was that it was due to "swelling" of the brain, but nothing definite was ever decided about it.

As the days passed and I remained in this dismal state, friends later told me they would sit and stare at my chest to see if I was still breathing. Some were making plans to check me out of the hospital so I could die peacefully at home. A "niece" from San Francisco who called one night to ask about my condition was told by the nurse in charge that I was worse, starting to have seizures, and was "an accident waiting to happen."

All I remember of this period were two dream/hallucinations, that still remain excruciatingly vivid.

In the first, I am in a small chamber, totally isolated and guarded by a burly woman who looks like a prison matron. I am begging her to *please* let me go home. She adamantly refuses. In desperation I softly, conspiratorially, ask, "Would five thousand dollars make a difference?" Apparently it does because I am released and the dream/hallucination ends.

In the second, I am standing on a tiny platform suspended over a seemingly bottomless abyss. I'm trembling with fear, feeling that any moment I may fall to my doom. This time I have a male guard keeping me from getting off the platform to safety. I frantically plead for him to have mercy and release me from this precarious perch. He is angered by my mounting hysteria. "I thought you were a nice lady," he says with disgust, "but now I see you're just a bitch." Since it worked once before and since I'm in a much more terrifying situation now, I up the ante. "Would ten thousand dollars make a difference?" Again it works, and I am allowed to leave the platform.

These two dream/hallucinations remain so vivid that even now I keep expecting the guards to show up demanding that their bribes be paid (but the hospital bills should easily be able to cover these comparatively small charges).

I will spare you further details of my decline and fall. What I'm here for is to show you—whether you've had a stroke or are caring for someone who has—how to play the sorry hand you were dealt and, perchance, to win.

PART 1

THE STROKEE CHRONICLES

1

The Science of Strokes

· · · · · · · · · · · · · · · · ·

A STROKE BY ANY OTHER NAME

One post-stroke problem you may have—albeit a very minor one—is deciding what to call yourself. "Stroke victim" has an ominous ring. "Stroke sufferer" is even worse. You don't want to have people believe that you are in constant agony; it's an even worse image to plant it in your own mind. "Stroke patient" isn't accurate for long since you're technically only a patient while you're in the hospital or rehab center or your doctor's office. "A person recovering from a stroke" is too cumbersome. "Stroke survivor" is as good as it gets since it conjures up an image of spunky Reba McEntire belting out a triumphant "I'm a survivor!"

Still, as one who doesn't like to leave well enough alone, thinking myself deucedly clever, I came up with the term "strokee." This is along the line of lessee—"a person to whom a lease is granted"—since, in a sense, you have received, or been granted, a stroke.

Then, when Barbara was browsing the Internet a little later on, to her surprise—and mine!—she came across the following "edi-tor's note" on the Web site www.strokesafe.org: "For the purposes of this manual, the terms 'survivor,' 'victim,' 'strokee,' and 'pa-tient' are interchangeable."

It may seem a bit strange to you now, but since, to conserve space and avoid confusion, we'll be using the term "strokee" throughout this book, you'll soon find it will trip easily off your tongue.

WHAT IS A STROKE?

A stroke occurs when the brain is deprived of blood. This can happen when a blood vessel has ruptured or, as is more common, is blocked by a clot. The lack of oxygen damages, or even kills, brain cells and disrupts functions controlled by the affected part of the brain. Because blood brings vital oxygen and nutrients to the brain, while simultaneously removing carbon dioxide and cel-lular waste, this deprivation can have devastating effects if not treated medically at once.

There are basically two major kinds of strokes: ischemic and hemorrhagic, along with subtypes that run the gamut from lacu-nar and cerebellar strokes to the so-called "silent stroke."

Ischemic Strokes

The most common type of stroke—comprising 85 percent of all strokes—is the ischemic stroke. This occurs when something (a blood clot, fatty material, or some other organic matter) blocks an artery leading to the brain and cuts off the supply of oxygen-bearing blood, thereby depriving the brain of the oxygen it needs to function properly.

Cerebellar Stroke
Located in the part of the brain on the lower backside of the skull, above the neck, the cerebellum controls balance and coordina-

tion. Symptoms of this kind of stroke can mimic those of vertigo or food poisoning—vomiting, dizziness, difficulty walking straight, etc. As with all strokes, immediate medical attention is extremely important to recovery.

Transient Ischemic Attack (TIA)

One common subtype of an ischemic stroke is a transient ischemic attack (TIA) (sometimes called "a mini stroke" or a "warning stroke"). This is usually very brief and not permanently damaging. Unlike a full-blown stroke, a TIA is a temporary interruption of blood flow to the brain when little bits of foreign matter lodge in small blood vessels in the brain. When this interrupts the flow of blood to an area of the brain, that area stops functioning until the bits of vascular rubble are dissolved. These episodes are brief, lasting from minutes to hours, with full recovery within twenty-four hours. They should not, however, be ignored: in the United States, more than a third of individuals who experience a TIA will have a stroke within five years.

Hemorrhagic Strokes

A hemorrhagic stroke occurs when a damaged or diseased blood vessel in the brain ruptures, resulting in bleeding in the brain. For obvious reasons, this is colloquially known as a "bleeder." Like most strokes, a hemorrhagic stroke is caused by high blood pressure. Compared to ischemic strokes, however, these kinds of events are relatively rare—only 12 percent of all strokes are of this type.

JUNE'S STROKES

My first stroke was hemorrhagic. About nine months later I had a much milder ischemic one; but since it occurred in exactly the same area of the brain as my first stroke, it wiped out the progress

Symptoms of a Stroke or TIA

Any or all of the below can be indicators of an impending stroke or one already in progress.

- Sudden numbness and weakness, especially in an arm or leg
- Garbled or slurred speech
- Confusion or difficulty comprehending speech
- Vision problems such as double vision or loss or diminished vision, often in one eye
- Poor coordination, staggering, or lack of balance sometimes resulting in a fall
- Unusually severe headaches with no other known cause (such as a preexisting migraine condition, etc.)
- Brief loss of consciousness
- Vomiting or nausea

I had made in physical and occupational therapy. I've also suffered several TIAs. The first one occurred several months prior to my major stroke and before I knew anything about stroke symptoms. Because I have diabetes, I assumed I was having an insulin reaction since the symptoms are similar to a stroke (although I was puzzled at the time because my blood sugar was normal).

When I first began experiencing TIAs, I'd call the paramedics to rush me to the hospital, which was only ten minutes away. Usually the symptoms disappeared while I was in the ambulance. But once a hospital has you in its clutches it's very difficult to extricate yourself, so I would spend the rest of the day in the emergency room, with occasional forays to other parts of the hospital to get a number of tests—MRI, EKG, etc. Even though none of the tests would show anything, I'd have to remain in the hospital overnight "just to be on the safe side." Much as I disliked the arduous and expensive TIA/hospital experience, the safe side is where I always want to be so I endured it.

I'm now in my fourth year of post-stroke living and it is, as the orphans' song from the musical *Annie* puts it, "a hard-knock life." And sometimes, you feel, just as the kids in the "orphanidge" felt, that your "life isn't worth a smidge." But all I can do—and all *you* can do—is confront your situation with the two sturdy lions who stand guard at the New York Public Library: Patience and Fortitude. They were named in the midst of the Great Depression by Mayor Fiorello LaGuardia because he said that's what you had to have to overcome the dismal economic situation at that time. Too, patience and fortitude will be what you need to have to confront *your* situation.

RISK FACTORS: WHY ME? WHY YOU? WHY DOES ANYBODY HAVE A STROKE?

Those of us who've already had a stroke will want to avoid any risk factors that might make us susceptible to another. There are two kinds of risk factors: the modifiable kind, those we have control over and, well, the other kind. Modifiable risk factors include:

High Blood Pressure (Hypertension)

High blood pressure is the number one risk factor for stroke. Keeping your blood pressure in the normal range is vital. It should consistently be at or under 140/90. Often you can control your blood pressure by losing weight and cutting back on your salt intake; but if that doesn't work for you, your doctor can prescribe a suitable medication with minimal side effects (see page 62).

In *The Diabetic's Total Health and Happiness Book* we point out that there are "furry blood pressure pills" that reduce your blood pressure with zero side effects: pets. Dr. Karen Allen, a professor at the University of Buffalo, presented a fascinating study at the March 1997 meeting of the American Psychosomatic Society. This study of one hundred women—half in their mid-twenties and the other half in their early seventies—showed that owning a pet can lower your blood pressure. Half the women in both age groups had a loved and loving cat or dog; the other half had never owned a pet. The women in each age group who had pets had lower blood pressure than those without pets. The blood pressure differences were the most dramatic in the older-women group. (For more on the value of pets to a strokee see "Fur-Covered Caregivers," page 28.)

High Cholesterol

As with most scientific research there is some controversy regarding studies about cholesterol. Is a high level of cholesterol a risk factor for heart attack and stroke, and does your diet influence that cholesterol level? Most studies indicate yes on both scores. But a minority of scientists maintain that those results are "inconclusive" in the matter of diet: Since the body manufactures its own cholesterol, they maintain, what you eat is not all that important. But as someone who has had strokes and wants to avoid more of the same, I'm voting with the majority.

Guidelines from the National Heart, Lung, and Blood Institute state that blood cholesterol should ideally fall below 200 milligrams. In the 200 to 239 range a person is at moderate risk for cardiovascular incidents. Levels of more than 240 puts a person at high risk. For those with cholesterol over 240, the institute recommends treatment first by diet and, if that fails, by medication.

In July 2004, the bad guys were further indicted by the National Institutes of Health, which reduced its recommended levels of LDL for those of moderately high risk to below 100. Higher than that, statins (cholesterol-lowering drugs) should be prescribed.

That's 30 points lower than the previous recommendation. For those with very high risk, the recommended level for cholesterol-lowering treatment drops to 70.

Over time, an elevated level of cholesterol can cause the blockage of blood vessels (atherosclerosis), a time honored and much-feared stroke risk. Postmenopausal women need to pay particular attention to their cholesterol. This is because women's estrogen levels decrease after menopause, and, as a result, their cholesterol levels increase. This can cause a buildup of arterial plaque and, as one thing leads to another, a greater stroke risk. One chilling statistic drives this point home: More than 60 percent of stroke deaths in the United States happen to postmenopausal women.

Diabetes

Diabetes can cause small blood vessels to close prematurely. When that happens to vessels in the brain, strokes may occur. There are two kinds of diabetes: type 1 and type 2. At this stage of medical science, you can't kick type 1 diabetes no matter how hard you—and the Juvenile Diabetes Foundation—try. Just ask the woman who's had type 1 for thirty-six years. But the good news is that you can control it; by keeping your blood sugar in the normal range you will greatly diminish your risk of a stroke.

Type 2 diabetes is another matter. This is the kind of diabetes that usually occurs later in life and is associated with obesity (along with the often concomitant sedentary lifestyle). In the United States, excess weight is reaching epidemic proportions. The most frightening—and previously unheard of— aspect is its appearance in children. There is even a term for the type of diabetes appearing in young people due to obesity: maturity-onset diabetes of the young (or MODY).) In July 2004, Medicare changed a longtime policy and recognized obesity as a disease.

This means Medicare will pay for weight-loss treatments for those diagnosed as obese (a body mass index above 30). This represents 18 percent of the Medicare population.

By eating a healthy diet, losing excess weight, and exercising more, you can control the effects of type 2 diabetes. While you can't technically *cure* your diabetes, you can virtually be symptom-free. That's the next best thing to not having diabetes at all.

For understanding diabetes and help in controlling or avoiding it, you might look inside one of our books on diabetes, particularly *The Diabetic's Book: All Your Questions Answered.*

Smoking

Smoking causes severe atherosclerosis—the buildup of plaques (deposits of fatty substances, cholesterol, calcium, etc.) on the lining of arteries, particularly the carotid. Not only do plaques grow large enough to reduce blood flow in an artery, but they can rupture, causing blood clots to form, further diminishing the flow of blood or—worse still—wandering off to a blood vessel that feeds the brain and blocking it, causing a stroke.

The doctors on the Web site www.MedicineNet.com put it bluntly: "When an individual smokes, the question becomes—which will occur first: a stroke, heart attack, or lung cancer?" So don't be an "eedjit" (the Irish version of idiot): Don't smoke!

Incidentally, when we went to Ireland several years back, we couldn't even go into pubs to hear the music and indulge in other publike activities because the smoke in the air there was so thick. But in 2004 the Irish gave up one major "eedjitism." They no longer allow smoking in pubs. *Erin Go Bragh!*

Atrial Fibrillation

The American Heart Association defines atrial fibrillation (AF) this way: "In it the heart's two small upper chambers (the atria) quiver instead of beating effectively. Blood isn't pumped completely out of them, so it may pool and clot. If a piece of a blood clot in the atria leaves the heart and becomes lodged in an artery in the brain, a stroke results." This is obviously a condition that calls for medical intervention. Coumadin, a blood thinner, is often prescribed and will require periodic checks to make sure it's doing the job. Note: Coumadin does increase a risk for internal or external bleeding.

PPA (Phenylpropanolamine)

Never heard of it? Neither had we until Sunday, March 28, 2004, when we opened the *Los Angeles Times* to find a shocking article by Kevin Sack and Alicia Mundy on the topic of PPA (for which they truly deserve a medal from the American Stroke Association). In it they tell of the drug industry's two-decade long struggle to keep cold medicines and diet drugs containing PPA on the store shelves despite the fact that since 1982 it was known that PPA could cause some people—most often young women—to suffer hemorrhagic strokes and other cardiovascular problems. In describing the PPA-related strokes of two of the young women, Sack and Mundy wrote: "Only hours before these devastating strokes, each victim had washed down a seemingly innocuous over-the-counter cold medicine, one of billions of doses consumed annually nationwide." The irony is that in their effort to keep these highly profitable products on the market, drug companies sponsored a five million dollar Yale University study to prove there was no link between PPA and strokes. But lo, the study showed the contrary—so the drug industry promptly launched a campaign to discredit the study.

The story is long and heartbreaking. It's one thing for a person of my age who has had a full life to be felled by a stroke, but quite another for it to happen to young women—and some men—who are just starting out. To have it happen as a result of corporate greed and deception is even more appalling. (The *Times* article points out that "more than 2,500 lawsuits have been filed by plaintiffs who say they suffered strokes shortly after taking products with PPA.")

PPA is no longer allowed in over-the-counter cough and cold medications and weight-loss products. But beware: if you're like many, you may have some products in your medicine cabinet that were purchased before the ban that you just left there in case you needed them later. If so, be sure to check and see if they contain PPA. Some brands that *previously* contained PPA are: Alka-Seltzer Plus, Comtrex, Contac, Triaminic, Tavist D, Acutrim, Dexatrim, Dimetapp, and Robitussin CF.

To read the entire *Los Angeles Times* article on PPA, titled "A Dose of Denial," check out www.latimes.com/ppa. To read the FDA's report on PPA, go to: www.fda.gov/cder/drug/infopage/ppa/default.htm.

Periodontitis (Advanced Gum Disease)

Here's a most surprising—even shocking—risk factor revealed by research from the State University of New York at Buffalo. Their study of nearly 10,000 people (aged twenty-five to seventy-five) showed that those who have severe gum disease run twice the risk for an ischemic stroke than those with healthy gums. Periodontitis is a bacterial infection that causes pockets to develop around the teeth. These pockets become a breeding ground for germs. The infection from the germ-laden gum pockets can cause bone and tooth loss and the infection can spread bacteria to other areas of the body. In addition, the bacteria in the pockets can make their way into the blood circulation, where it can wreak havoc on the linings of the arteries. These bacteria can also lead to clotting, possibly causing strokes.

A consistent and healthy dental program, while important for everyone, is very important for stroke survivors. They should be particularly diligent in taking care of their teeth. Loss of some sensation, weakness in jaw and facial muscles, and even certain medications can put you at an elevated risk for periodontitis—increasing your risk for stroke.

Constipation

This is really the low man on the stroke risk totem pole, but take it from me: If it leads to "straining at stool," it can result in a stroke of the serious hemorrhagic kind. If constipation is a problem for you, see "Conquering Constipation" on page 71.

Patent Foramen Ovale (PFO)

More and more, doctors are encountering younger people who suffer strokes because of a defect in the heart called a patent foramen ovale, or a small hole in the heart, located in the atrial septum. This hole exists in everyone before birth. It is utilized during fetal circulation to help faciliate travel of blood through the heart (this is because in the womb, babies do not use their own lungs for oxygen-rich blood). Typically, this hole closes at birth when blood pressure on the left side of the heart forces the opening closed. However, in many people, this doesn't happen, and the result is a defect called a PFO. Usually, it doesn't cause a problem. It works like a flap valve, only opening when there is more pressure in the chest area than usual. However, increased pressure can heighten risk for a stroke—and this pressure can come from violent coughing, vomiting, straining at stool, or even a vigorous sneeze. If the pressure is severe enough, blood moves from the right atrium to the left atrium, and if there happens to be a clot, or even particles in the blood, traveling in the right side, it can force its way through the PFO and find its way to the brain, causing a stroke.

The PFO can be treated with heart surgery or a cardiac implant. Unfortunately, though, the PFO is usually only discovered *after* a stroke or heart attack caused by the defect. You may

ask your doctor about this at your annual exam. More information can be found at the Adult Congenital Heart Association Web
site: www.achaheart.org.

Dangerous Drugs

On September 30, 2004, Vioxx, the arthritis and acute pain relief
medication—and the largest-selling prescription drug in history—
was taken off the market. A new study had revealed a higher rate
of heart attacks and strokes among patients taking that drug than
among those taking a placebo. Options being considered to replace
Vioxx include Celebrex and Bextra (both COX-2 inhibitors, like
Vioxx) and certain over-the-counter pain drugs. If you are making
changes to your pain medications, it is imperative that you discuss
these changes with your doctor and also that you remain alert to
reports of new drug studies.

Catching a Stroke in the Neck of Time

When there is a blockage in the carotid artery in the neck, the clot
can break loose and travel quickly to the brain, causing a stroke.
That is why carotid artery scans are frequently given to people with
a history of strokes. I have had two of these scans, neither of which
revealed a blockage. But when a blockage is found, until recently it
was necessary to cut into the neck and artery, remove the blockage,
and stitch the artery and neck back up. This procedure required
general anesthesia and hospitalization of up to four days.

But now the FDA has approved a stent (a "balloon" catheter—
small expandable tube) and filter system that can remove the blockage without such an invasive procedure. The stent is inserted into an
incision in the groin and sent up through the artery into the neck.
The balloon catheter then expands to dislodge the blockage, which
is then caught in the filter and removed, thereby preventing a stroke.

At this time, the FDA has approved the use of the stent and filter system in those with high risk patients with 80 percent or
greater blockage, but the manufacturer is currently conducting
clinical trials to prove that it is as safe as surgery for lower-risk
patients. They expect the trials will be completed in 2007 or
2008, and if they prove that the procedure is as safe as surgery in
lower-risk patients, then they will ask the FDA for approval for
use in all patients with carotid blockages.

DIFFERENT STROKES FOR DIFFERENT FOLKS

The basic principle of strokes is that no two are *exactly* alike. The
physical and/or mental damage to your mind and/or body is your
own particular configuration of losses or changes. The rate at
which you improve may be faster or slower than other people.

For instance, my mind still works—or I couldn't be writing this
book. Since Barbara is so frequently overwhelmed by a combination
of her many old and new responsibilities, she tends to lose her focus
and her mind gets a bit muddled. We like to say that if we put
together my mind and her body, we'd have one really good person.

Location, Location, Location!

Just as in real estate, the most important factor in a stroke is the
location. The part of the brain where the stroke occurs controls
the functions of the opposite side of the body. A stroke in the
right hemisphere of the brain affects the left side; one in the left
hemisphere affects the right. Along with that, there are other variations in functions depending on which area of the brain has been
damaged. The following are some of the possible effects of a
stroke, depending on in which hemisphere and in which part of
that hemisphere suffered the stroke.

Cerebellar Stroke

The cerebellum is located in the lower back of the brain, just above the brainstem. If only one of the two hemispheres of the cerebellum has suffered a stroke, *the same side of the body will be affected rather than the opposite.* Effects of a stroke in the cerebellum may include:

• Loss of balance, the person may seem drunk: staggering, walking with feet wide apart, wobbling and weaving
• Slurred speech
• Poor muscular coordination, shaking of the extremities (ataxia)
• Rapid flickering side-to-side eye movement (nystagmus)

JUNE'S STROKE II

The good news is that one rarely develops all of the possible problems associated with whatever kind of stroke one had. For example, because my stroke took place in the left hemisphere of my brain, it caused some paralysis (particularly in the hand and arm and leg) of the right side of my body (right hemiplegia). I'm extremely right-handed, so this posed a problem with writing, eating, and doing all the things I formerly did with my right hand. (Once when I was having physical therapy there was a woman in the rehab area who had had a stroke in her right hemisphere, which meant her left side was affected and her right side unimpaired. "Boy, are you lucky," I said enviously. "Not so lucky," she said. "I'm left-handed.")

Although a left-hemisphere stroke sometimes causes aphasia (problems with speech and writing and reading), I managed to escape that. I'm able to talk, but when I'm tired—as I often am—my speech gets slurry with my words a little chewed-up sounding.

Reading is no problem, except that with only one usable hand, it's hard to turn the pages of a book and near impossible to turn the pages of a newspaper. Of course with my chronic right-handedness, writing is a problem. I now print with my left hand. If I were a second grader I'd probably get a D in that skill or, if I had a very forgiving teacher, maybe a C–.

When I'm tired I don't swallow well on the right side of my throat, and that makes me choke easily. The most annoying and embarrassing aspect of my strokes is one many other strokees complain about: We have a tendency to drool on the stroke-struck side, especially when eating. It's not that it's as bad as a cocker spaniel watching the preparations for his dinner. It's more like a little pearl forming in the corner of my mouth which, if not blotted away, turns into a rivulet and starts to trickle chinward.

I've not been able to drive since my stroke, but that is not as great a loss as you might think. As an insulin-taking diabetic, I worried about my pre-stroke driving anyway, because I knew that if I should have a low blood sugar incident, I wouldn't be the safest thing on wheels.

There are many things I can't do now, or can't do as well as I once did. But I try not to blight my days by mourning over the losses, and neither should you. It's better just to kiss them good-bye, make the necessary adaptations, and move on.

The violinist Itzhak Perlman once broke a string in the middle of a piece he was playing in a concert. Without missing a beat he continued on to the end, transposing the piece onto the three remaining strings. When people complimented him on his feat, he said, smiling, "It's good to see what you can do with what you've got left." This statement had particular significance for him since he had polio as a child and lost the use of his legs—and it has particular significance for *you*.

Left Hemisphere Stroke	Right Hemisphere Stroke
• Right side paralysis and/or weakness	• Left side paralysis and/or weakness
• Loss of vision on the right side	• Loss of vision on the left side
• Difficulty in speaking and/or understanding	• Slurred speech
• Difficulty in reading and/or writing	• Difficulty with eating and swallowing
• Difficulty in working with numbers	• Depression and mood swings
	• Poor memory and sense of time

CHAPTER 2

After the Stroke

· · · · · · · · · · · · · · · · · · ·

There is no good arguing with the inevitable. The only argument available with an east wind is to put on your overcoat.

— JAMES RUSSELL LOWELL, *Democracy and Other Addresses*

Brace yourself. You may have some unexpected—and unwelcome— experiences after your stroke. Try not to let them get to you. They're inevitable. The only thing you can do is put on your emotional overcoat and weather the buffeting winds.

COPING WITH THE INEVITABLES OF A STROKE

Coming Home

One inevitable you're going to be facing is a happy one: returning home from your hospital or rehab center stay. But not so happy is the fact that you've changed and, as a result, your home is going to need some changing. Before you're released you should have a meeting with your physical and occupational therapists and the institution's social worker. They have a lot of experience in helping strokees adjust to the return and helping the house adjust to the new you.

Things you will need to consider:

- You may need to buy or rent a hospital bed, or at least an electric one. This will help not only you, but your home caregiver who may, depending upon the severity of your stroke, have to help you in and out of bed.
- Any toilet you will be using will likely need an elevated seat.
- If you have been using a wheelchair, you will need to have one at home—or maybe two: one standard wheelchair for home and a light-weight transport one for going to the doctor, out to lunch or dinner or the movies or theater or shopping. If you plan to do work at a desk or table or want to be able to draw near to the dining table—and you probably will—be sure to get a desk wheelchair. This is the kind that has arms that are lower in front, the better to slip under things.
- You should have easy access to a phone, so you will need a phone jack near your bed or, better still, a cell phone or portable phone, which you can also use to summon your caregiver when he or she is out.

Just visualize your home situation and try to remember what tools, pieces of furniture, and other items you use most in your everyday domestic life. Then make sure they will be accessible when you get home. Consider especially the kitchen and what you intend to be doing there.

HOME NURSES, HELPERS, AND CAREGIVERS

One challenging yet unavoidable aspect of stroke recovery is the question of caregiving. Even those of us who have suffered the mildest of strokes will require some immediate help—and the majority of strokees will need some longer-term care. This care will be specific to the strokee's needs because, as I mentioned at the outset of the book, each stroke is unique. There are, unfortunately, some difficult issues awaiting you and your caregiver during this time, including navigating the tangled web that is health insurance coverage and finding a suitable home nurse or caregiver from an agency. But with a little knowledge—and the Web addresses and phone numbers of some of the numerous patient advocacy groups and stroke associations—you will be well-armed to face the fray!

Custodial Care Catch-22

First the bad news: When it comes to home nurses and other non-family caregivers, you're pretty much on your own. This is why most home care is done *pro bono* by family members and friends. I have health insurance from a company that, for anonymity's sake, we'll call "Double Cross." It's actually pretty good coverage—although, as with many insurance companies, the benefits erode and co-pays increase each year. However, my insurance paid for absolutely no home care after my stroke, despite the fact that the list of benefits that were covered under the plan included "Home Health Care—100% up to 100 visits per 12-month period."

There is another culprit (for those who rely on Medicare), outside of the individual insurance agencies—the federal government. The Balanced Budget Act of 1997 reduced reimbursement to agencies that provide Medicare services. Rehabilitation hospitals are now reducing the number of Medicare patients they accept due to lower reimbursements. In addition, home health agencies are also reducing services for the same reason.

From the moment I was released from the hospital, I needed

help with things such as blood sugar tests and blood pressure checks, insulin injections, bathing, dressing, bathroom visits, and so on. Feeling that the insurance company would be more likely to pay if the home care was provided by an official agency rather than a handpicked private caregiver, I hired one from an agency the hospital recommended. My theory, however, proved to be wrong.

Dealing with insurance companies may prove at times to be as challenging as rehabilitating your body. It's an unfortunate fact of life that you will have to deal with, and will require persistence and patience. Even though Barbara, the most persistent of creatures, bombarded my insurance company with letters and documentation, she got nowhere in her quest for reimbursement. A typical letter of hers read this way[1]:

To Whom It May Concern:

Acting as June Biermann's patient advocate, I want to explain to you the circumstances that cause Mrs. Biermann to require home health care. Not only did the stroke, which she suffered on July 10, affect her right leg, arm, and hand (she is very right-handed) but she has been a type 1 (insulin-requiring) diabetic for thirty-three years and now has high blood pressure. She is currently not able to test her blood sugar, which must be done as often as seven times a day, measure and inject her insulin, which must be done a minimum of five times a day, and check her blood pressure once a day.

Medicare only briefly provides the services of a visiting nurse. In the beginning the nurse came every other day, and then only for a brief period, usually around an hour. Then it was reduced to three times a week, and now she no longer comes at all. Actually,

[1]See the section on patient advocacy in part 2, page 190.

*the one blood sugar test and the blood pressure test she took were
far from adequate for Mrs. Biermann's home care needs.*

*I have enclosed the records from the home care agency providing
the nurses to show the services that were rendered and the costs
thereof. If you need further explanation or documentation don't
hesitate to contact me.*

Barbara never heard a word from the insurance company. When
she called the company to see what was going on she talked to a
nice woman who said she would check on the situation. Barbara
never heard from her either, so she started calling her back again
and again. Finally Barbara learned their decision: They determined
that I was receiving "custodial care," and insurance does not pay for
custodial care. Case closed.

Barbara browsed the Internet under "custodial care." She found
the term generally defined as: "Helps a person perform 'activities
of daily living,' which include assistance with eating, bathing,
etc."; "Usually given by people without medical skills"; "Less
intensive and complicated than skilled or intermediate care"; "Can
be provided in many different settings, including nursing homes,
adult day care centers, or at home"; "Sometimes custodial care is
called 'personal care.'"

All right. But what if the person *has* medical skills and uses
them, as in my case, to test blood sugar, and inject insulin, and
take blood pressure, then occasionally delivers a plate of food or
assists the patient in going to the bathroom or helps the patient
in or out of bed?

The Internet is full of cases of people trying (and failing!) to
get insurance companies to pay for what they unilaterally decree
as "custodial care." So I was not alone.

Late-Breaking News

On the last Health Benefits Program I received from my insurance company, I discovered that they had totally eliminated *all* home care benefits. Actually it's better that they should eliminate a benefit that they never pay than one that they actually promised to pay on a benefits list. That way they can also save more money by laying off the employees who handle the claims for home health care benefits and just respond to each query from caregivers and strokees: "This is custodial care and insurance does not pay for custodial care."

On the Internet we found a remark concerning Champus (the Civilian Health and Medical Program for the Uniformed Services). It said that Champus "uses its definition in a strange way, as if to say that if the patient needs assistance with 'activities of daily living' (ADLs in medical jargon), all care that the patient receives, even if it admittedly falls within the Champus definition of 'skilled nursing care,' is excluded from coverage on the premise that it is 'custodial care.'"

Probably a few years back I should have taken out long-term care insurance. And then again, maybe not. As Stephen M. Pollan wrote in his book *Die Broke:* "I really want to be able to tell you to take out long-term care insurance as soon as possible . . . but I can't . . . the industry is a snake pit of lying salesmen, onerous provisions obscured by arcane language, fly-by-night insurers looking to make a quick buck, and horror stories that are all too common. There's little federal or state regulation or control over the business, and what few rules are in place are hardly ever enforced. It really is a disgrace."

It is to be hoped that some governmental regulation or control will be imposed to correct this. But in the meantime if you want to be sure that you have someone to care for you when you need it and for as long as you need it, you have a couple of options:

1. Win the lottery.
2. Be really, *really* nice to your family and friends so you can rely on their help.

Often it happens that one kindhearted family member takes on the entire burden of caregiving while the others living too far away or claiming too many family responsibilities of their own get by with occasional cards and visits on special occasions. Barbara had a friend who cared for her invalid mother for years while holding down a job as a librarian. Her sister, who lived out of town, was seldom if ever seen until the mother died. Then the sister immediately appeared and demanded her half of the estate, including the house that had been promised to the librarian, who had done all the caregiving for her mother.

This kind of thing happens frequently enough to make it imperative that any arrangement in which something is promised in exchange for caregiving should be written up in an unbreakable legal document (see Part 2). You can get some guidance in this by looking up "legal documents for caregivers" in a search engine on the Internet. If, however, it's a matter of a house or large estate, it's wise to consult an attorney, especially if there are relatives waiting in the wings.

Another development in the caregiving scene was reported by *The Wall Street Journal* a couple of years ago. This involves paying a family member, who could not otherwise afford to do it, to provide care. The other family members can share the cost or, if the disabled person has funds, the payment could come from that— or later be paid from his or her estate. In some states, Medicaid programs are now allowing disabled persons to employ family members rather than home care agencies as caregivers.

Helpful Resources

- American Stroke Association: www.strokeassociation.com, 1-888-478-7653
- National Stroke Association: www.stroke.org, 1-800-STROKES
- Patient Advocate Foundation: www.patientadvocate.org, 1-800-532-5274
- College of American Pathologists' helpful Web site on managing the maze of health care: www.cap.org/apps/docs/fact_sheets/maze.htm

CAREGIVERS: THE BAD AND THE BEAUTIFUL

Since getting out of the hospital after my initial stroke in 2000, I have had five caregivers. The first one, sent by the agency, was totally unreliable. She was always late and always wanted to leave early because she had her own importing business on the side. She didn't last long. The second one, also from the agency, was competent and professional and took good care of my medical needs. But that is all she did, except crochet baby blankets for a charitable organization. A noble calling, but I could have used a little more custodial care from her. This woman finally had to leave me because she got a better job working full time for a one-hundred-year-old woman who wanted live-in help. But she did do me a great favor: she was from the Philippines and recommended a friend from there to fill her position. (She turned out to be caregiver number three.) The new caregiver was also very competent in her nursing duties and was especially good at such "custodial" activities as cleaning out things and reorganizing. She was, in fact, a cleaning dervish. But, she didn't last very long either because her husband had a good job, and he wanted her there waiting for him when he got home.

Fortunately there is a huge network of Filipino people, many of them trained in nursing; so, before she left she recommended another woman from the Philippines. Unfortunately, she had only been with us a couple of weeks when she was called back home to the Phillipines for an emergency. But that turned out to be the best thing that ever happened to us because she had a daughter-in-law who could fill in for her. Number five was our lucky number. She was—and is—a wonder woman. Her name is Josefa, but her family called her Deding and so did we because she quickly became like one of the family. She is extremely well-trained, a CNA, in fact—a certified nursing assistant. Deding does everything I need to have done for me and does it really well because she is so experienced. She is charming and cheerful and she also loves cleaning house as well as working in the garden. We love her. She's been with us over three years now and we hope she never leaves.

However, we do have to pay for her caregiving out of pocket. There was, in our case, truly no alternative. And thereby hangs the tale of why most people have to rely on the kindness of relatives. In my case, both Barbara and Deding are caregivers. In the beginning, Barbara did all the caregiving, but gradually, to preserve both Barbara's health and her sanity, Deding has taken on more and more responsibility

In addition, you can see from all we went through to find Deding that it's not easy to find a good caregiver, let alone a perfect one. But it's worth the effort to persevere until you find your own wonderful caregiver, if you're hiring someone from outside the family. In your search, it is vital that you make a list for yourself of the qualities you consider most important in a caregiver. Some general traits to look for in your quest include:

- nursing skills
- compatibility

- kindness
- common sense and intelligence (the former is more important than the latter!)
- reliability
- a sense of humor (vital for us!)
- energy—and the willingness to expend that energy whenever and wherever it's needed
- and, most of all, that *je ne sais quoi,* that ineffable something that lets you know he or she is "The One"

Seek and you shall find.

Fur-Covered Caregivers

Several years ago when I had my broken leg (or shattered tibial plateau, to make it sound as serious as it was) I discovered that there is no caregiver who can equal a pet caregiver. (Sorry about that, Barbara.) My cat Lucy stayed on my bed giving cat comfort twenty-four hours a day for two solid weeks until the worst was over. Only then would she resume her normal feline activities. She still always checked in on me several times a day. All this attention was given without a penny of monetary recompense or a word of complaint.

In most cases, a dog would do as well as a cat, but in a stroke situation, especially when you have weakness or hemiplegia (paralysis on one side) a dog wouldn't be advised since one of their great joys is to have you take them for walks. A dog tugging mightily on a leash could easily topple an unsteady person. I recently read that cats are recommended to AIDS patients for the same reason. Dogs—unlike Lucy and her fellow felines—are not content to stay put on your bed or lap. They are more likely to keep poking you with an insistent paw or bark their desire to go out or pathetically hold a leash in their mouths.

Cats can also manage their natural needs with a litter box that can be cleaned daily by the human caregiver. (Just what every caregiver needs—another task to perform.)

FATIGUE AND EXHAUSTION

Every stroke-recovering person I know suffers from and is baffled by their fatigue/exhaustion. Dorothy, a New York friend who had a stroke a couple of years before mine, e-mailed us: "I'm okay but very tired. I need to take time off from work for a while, but a college education for two kids is too expensive for me to do that." She says that often at the end of the work day when she walks through the office and colleagues call to her to chat about something, she just waves and walks on by because she knows that in her state of fatigue her speech wouldn't be up to its usual snuff, and they might have difficulty understanding her.

Once when she and her children signed up for a litter clean-up day sponsored by their church, she reported later, "Yes, I had my litter clean-up day. It put me back two weeks. I try to do something meaningful and I get wiped out."

I know how she feels. My energy suddenly gives out and I have to lie down. This just isn't typical June behavior. Put the blame on the strokee within. My advice is to listen to your body, even if you don't want to. Your body knows best, and really, there's no other choice.

One warning, though: Your family and friends will probably have difficulty understanding this, especially if you've been a hyper-energetic person all your life. Explain to them that this is a good thing, a natural thing. It's just your body focusing on healing itself. A nurse friend of mine says that animals know this. When they are sick or injured they go off by themselves and sleep more. Another friend, who had four years of graduate study in biology at Harvard, compared the post-stroke situation to travel in a foreign country. She says you have to rest and sleep more than usual because the brain is working so hard processing new experiences that it gets exhausted. The same holds true for babies. Practically everything that happens to them is a new experience and they need that sleep time for the brain to digest it.

The brain of a person who's had a stroke may be creating new pathways, which, in a sense, are like new experiences. So it's tiring— *very* tiring. Even reading, which may have been something you whiled away an afternoon enjoying in the past, may become a bit taxing, especially if you're a history buff or a fan of other types of nonfiction. If you find that reading tuckers you out, take little breaks, but definitely don't put down your books indefinitely. Reading can help you recover.

Many physical therapists don't understand this tiredness—or won't accept it. They keep pressing you to do more. That's not too surprising. After all, that's their job, and they want you to make progress. Back when I had shattered my tibial plateau, my orthopedist cautioned me that therapists often tend to be too aggressive in their treatments and I should be careful not to let them push too hard. There's a delicate balance between giving your all to do what the therapist wants, even if it feels like too much for you, and giving up at the first twinge of discomfort or fatigue. All you can do is try to do your best.

EMOTIONS

You'll also be surprised at your loss of emotional control. The Koreans even have a term for it—emotional incontinence! You may find yourself crying for no reason whatsoever; you may not even be feeling sad at the time. This will be shocking to you—and to others!—especially if you have always been the opposite of a crybaby type. What to do? I say just let it flow. It will stop in due time, again for no reason whatsoever. When I was at the rehab center, the staff often provided entertainment in the afternoon, usually musicians and singers. Sometimes I would start crying over the songs they performed, even when the tunes were something as nonsentimental as "Oh Susanna" or "Row, Row, Row Your Boat."

Many stroke survivors have inexplicable, almost hysterical, laughing episodes. I think one of those would be a joy both to me and to those around me, but, alas, I have never experienced one. Katherine Sherwood, artist and art professor at the University of California, Berkeley, and strokee (see her fascinating story in "Other People's Strokes," page 201) has it both ways, emotionally speaking. She reports bursting into tears in the midst of a routine faculty meeting and laughing until her sides hurt while trying to discipline her daughter.

In February 2004, the *Los Angeles Times* reported that a new drug called Neurodex has been shown to reduce inappropriate emotional outbursts in people with brain injuries and neurological diseases (multiple sclerosis, Alzheimer's disease, Lou Gehrig's disease, Parkinson's disease, and, what we're particularly concerned with, strokes). It is estimated that the condition, called the pseudobulbar effect, is seen in 11 percent of people who have had a stroke. Regaining emotional stability is extremely important for strokees. Otherwise they may become withdrawn, hesitating to go out into the community because they fear having an embarrassing attack of "emotional incontinence."

Depression

My emotions and those of other stroke survivors tend to run to spells of depression. These depressive episodes are to be expected, what with such intense changes in your life. Some forms of depression are exaggerated forms of the normal emotional response to loss. In other words, it is melancholy writ large. And isn't that exactly how you feel and have every right to feel, especially at first, when the full impact of your situation hits you?

What has happened is that much of your life as you knew it has died along with those cells in your brain. One of the greatest losses we can suffer is a loss of a part of ourselves, not to mention the freedom to come and go and do what you please, when you please. Beautiful spontaneity! Who wouldn't mourn its loss? And you finally receive that most dire of warnings: you are not immortal.

How do you work through this kind of grief, which is overlaid with fear? You can't just pretend it's not there or suppress it. As Ovid said, "Suppressed grief suffocates." If you acknowledge your grief, you will pass through a mourning process not unlike what you would pass through at the death of a loved one, because in a very real sense, you have lost a very much loved one—your former self.

Most of us don't complete these steps in a rigid and logical order. No, it's more often a sloppier, random pattern. For instance, you may be angry first. Others start out with depression. You may swing back and forth from one stage to another, skipping some, repeating others, stagnating in still others.

I had a rather odd pattern. Since I wasn't expected to live after my first stroke, I started off with acceptance, an "I'm lucky to be alive" attitude. I think I had the feeling that with the miracle of survival, more miracles would surely follow. The improvement brought about by my early physical and occupational therapies reinforced my optimistic outlook. But nine months later, when I experienced the second stroke that wiped out all my progress and made me realize that I might never achieve my dreams of recovery, I jumped onto the Kübler-Ross roller coaster of mourning,

Mourning for Your Lost Self

Note: the following steps in **italics** are those of Kübler-Ross.* The augmentations are ours.

Elisabeth Kübler-Ross describes in *Death and Dying* the stages of the mourning process:

Denial *"This can't be happening to me. It will go away."*

Anger *In the perfectly justifiable anger at your situation, you often express it in the perfectly unjustifiable anger directed at those who are trying to help and care for you and who are doing the best they can in a difficult—or in some cases almost impossible—situation.*

Bargaining *In the case of someone who has had a stroke, you might bargain for the return of some of your lost powers and abilities: "If I could just use my right hand again, I promise I will . . ." or " If I could walk a mile unassisted, I swear I will never again . . ."*

Depression *Having come to the realization that the return of those lost or diminished powers and abilities may not be immediate or even imminent, you may grow melancholy and feel hopeless, believing that a "new you" is a "worse you."*

Acceptance *After a period of depression, you will have come to grips with the reality of your new situation, and a return of hope and energy may brighten your mood and give you new life.*

back and forth, one stage after the other. And I have been having a bumpy ride on and off ever since.

Now when I'm in a down mood I sometimes ask myself, "Where is the person of yesteryear?" Quoting the French *"Où*

---

*Dr. Elisabeth Kübler-Ross died on August 25, 2004, at the age of seventy-eight. She had been in declining health since a series of strokes in 1995. A firm believer in life after death, she was looking forward to meeting such personal idols as Gandhi and Carl Jung. After slipping off the bindings of illness, she said, "I'm going to dance in all the galaxies."

sont les neiges d'antan?" (Where are the snows of yesteryear?) But that's only when I'm feeling exceptionally bleak. Usually I count my blessings and not my bummers.

However, there are times when you should stop your bullet-biting and seek professional help for your feelings of depression. Even Barbara, who has always been almost a pathological optimist, finally sought counseling after trying—and failing—to overcome the depression that engulfed her during the first two years after my stroke. There is no shame in seeking psychological help, and it may even be the responsible thing for you to do, seeing as your moods and depressions affect another indispensable human being—your caregiver.

SETBACKS

Setbacks are not necessarily inevitable. They do happen, though, and it's best to be prepared for them. Setbacks can be physical or emotional, and you should be gentle with yourself when they occur. Most of the time, they are not of your making. And just because I've had a couple setbacks doesn't mean you will. I hope you won't, but if you *should,* just try to hang in there until you turn a corner into a happier place.

June's Setback #1

Nine months after my first stroke, I suffered a setback. Up until then I'd been chugging along and making great progress in my stroke recovery; but then in the middle of the night I found my right leg was so weak, I could hardly stand on it. In addition, my right arm had resumed the rigid spastic position (elbow bent, hand on heart). I thought it was just fatigue setting in after an unusually active day. The next day I took it easy, but still the weakness and spastic position remained. I decided something should be done.

At six the next morning, Barbara took me to the ER. After a great deal of waiting the staff took a CAT scan of my brain, but could see nothing. (As I mentioned previously, my first stroke had had a visible bleeding area about the size of a quarter.) The neurologist came in and did a few tests ("How many fingers do you see?" "Can you wiggle your toes?"). He couldn't find anything wrong either. The only thing left to do was to administer an MRI. When the results were returned, the doctor discovered an infarct of a small blood vessel in the area of my brain where the previous stroke had occurred. So this *was* a stroke, but a much milder one than the previous one—a "dry stroke" rather than a "bleeder."

They only kept me in the hospital for two days and one night, whereas with the first stroke I was "incarcerated" for three to four weeks. I was told to go home, take a baby aspirin every day, and resume my normal activities. Easier said than done, because the bad news was that this second stroke erased most of the progress I'd made over the course of nine months in physical and occupational therapy.

It was back to square one. It was going to take much more therapy and many more months before I'd be back to the point that I could "resume my normal activities."

June's Setback #2

In the autumn of my fourth year post-stroke, I experienced another setback. One morning at breakfast I felt strange and asked Barbara if she could help me eat. Barbara was baffled: "Help you eat? June, it's a soft-boiled egg. You don't need help with *that!*" But since I apparently just sat there looking pathetic, Barbara relented and was starting to spoon the egg into my mouth when I was hit with a bone-rattling seizure that Barbara said was even more frightening than one of my strokes.

Barbara called the paramedics, but when they arrived they

refused to take me to the hospital where my doctor practices; county protocol, they said, required them to take patients requiring emergency care to the closest hospital. The closest hospital in this case turned out to be a hospital Barbara thoroughly loathes— her father died there—and it has a much-deserved dismal reputation. I was in intensive care there for a few days for observation of the seizure's aftereffects, and then was transferred to the regular floor.

An aside: One morning Barbara arrived to find me lying quietly with my eyes closed. Next to my bed, a priest was saying prayers rather loudly. Thinking that I must be dying—or worse— Barbara dashed to the nurse's station to find out what disaster had befallen me. Everyone there seemed relaxed and unworried, so Barbara calmed down and asked one of the nurses what was going on with the priest. "Oh, don't worry about it," the nurse said. "Nothing's wrong. That's just Father X. He's retired and he drops by from time to time to pray with the patients. "

Having something to laugh about in a situation like this is invaluable. Those humorous moments are tough to find, but being overly somber does not necessarily add to a strokee's comfort when she's in a hospital bed. One funny moment for Barbara and me came when I had been scheduled for an MRI and Barbara was filling out a questionnaire for me before they could perform the test. Her favorite questions were: "Do you have a war injury or gunshot wound?" "Are you pregnant or nursing an infant?" and "Do you have any concealed body piercing?"

Strokes and Seizures

Seizures are one of the brain's responses to injury. They are also something that many stroke victims experience post-stroke. While a seizure is frightening for both patient and observer, they usually last only a few minutes and are rarely life-threatening, unless associated with a hazardous situation, such as swimming, bathing, driving, or a fall. You should tell your caregiver about this last point. Although a seizure is not to be taken lightly and an immediate trip to the hospital is definitely in order, caregivers should remain calm, assured that the situation is not as bad as it looks.

Dilantin

I had a seizure in conjunction with an earlier stroke, but it was no bone-rattler; in fact, the seizure was so mild that I didn't even know I'd had one. At that time my doctor gave me Dilantin, but took me off the drug when I recovered from the effects of the stroke and was sent home. I later learned that I shouldn't have been taken off Dilantin, because people who have suffered a hemorrhagic stroke are almost twice as likely to have a seizure than those who had ischemic strokes (now they tell me!). I was put back on Dilantin. Now I have my Dilantin level checked every two weeks to make sure it's high enough to prevent future seizures. Be sure to talk to your doctor about whether or not seizure medications are right for you post-stroke.

3

Recovery

. . . .

THE BASIC THERAPIES: OCCUPATIONAL, PHYSICAL, AND SPEECH

Therapy usually starts while you're still in the hospital. You may not be able to believe how quickly they want to get you up and at 'em. It's important that you cooperate and give your best effort. The sooner you do, the faster will be your progress on the bumpy road to recovery. There may be many roads available to you for rehabilitation, but the one you take is dependent upon a number of factors: severity of the stroke, your tolerance and stamina, insurance coverage, your financial situation, and even your geographical location. However, in general, your options for rehabilitation activities may include the rehabilitation unit in the hospital, an independent rehabilitation center, home therapy, outpatient therapy, and adult day services.

You will also have a whole cast of characters to become acquainted with: your physician; a neurologist (or a rehabilitative neurologist), who will assess your level of disability; and of course your rehab nurses, who will instruct you regarding medications, treatment, daily living activities, and any number of issues that will crop up for both the strokee and the caregiver.

After you've had what the hospital and your insurance company deem sufficient therapy, you are sent home. You may then go into home therapy, and when you graduate from that, to outpatient therapy in a hospital or rehabilitation facility. For home and out-patient therapy you will need a prescription from your physician in order to have it covered by Medicare or private insurance, or both.

Occupational Therapy

Despite its name, occupational therapy (OT) has nothing to do with getting you back to the office after the stroke. Occupational therapy has to do with such things as getting in and out of bed, usually completed without much thought in our pre-stroke days. It also deals with any kind of communication, such as writing, phoning, tape recording, or using a computer. Basically, OT helps the things you do everyday with the upper body (arms and hands mainly.)

There's another important task that an occupational therapist may be called upon to perform for you: preventing or treating shoulder subluxation. This is a condition in which the shoulder joint slides partially out of place. In strokees who have hemiplegia—paralysis of one arm—it's quite common (in fact, estimates can range from 17 percent of all stroke victims to 81 percent!).

I had and, alas, still have an extreme dislocation. The bone in the back of my shoulder sticks out and my arm hangs down from my shoulder and doesn't seem as well-connected as it once was. It has periods of being quite painful.

This subluxation can be a result of a weakening of muscles, improper positioning of the arm, or tugging on your stroke arm by caregivers, therapists, or other hospital personnel when they make transfers (moving you in and out of wheelchairs, on and off beds or examining tables, in and out of cars, etc.). This is something for you to watch for. Insist that you should always wear a gait belt when you are being lifted or moved around by anyone. (Also called a "transfer belt," a gait belt is a sturdy two-inch-wide web belt with a metal safety buckle closure for your helper to have something to hold onto and lift with.)

Subluxation can be treated by electrical stimulation, slings, and biofeedback. As with all stroke therapies, the sooner it's done, the more effective it will be. Some people find relief with biofeedback treatment and/or electrical stimulation of the shoulder muscle. Others use slings, cuffs, or arm troughs (there is debate about which of these is most effective). Do whatever is most comfortable and convenient for you.

When I first went home I had a visiting occupational therapist. He, to put it bluntly, was a bust. He was always late and often canceled. When he did show up, about all he did was run an electronic massaging device over my arm and shoulder and tap my arm while he kept a running narration of his life and career ambitions. I noticed no improvement as a result of his therapy, so I called the office to see if there was another occupational therapist available. There was and she was perfection: prompt, always "keeping on task" (the task of my therapy!) using many new (to me!) therapeutic techniques and skills, and on top of everything she was a nice person to have around. I feel I made great progress with her. Remember: the squeaking strokee gets the better therapists. Agencies are loath to lose a patient!

Physical Therapy

Physical therapy is usually shortened to PT, which some jocular patients like to say stands for "pain and torture." It is true that this is the most arduous of the therapy triumvirate. The physical therapist's area of operations is your lower body, legs, and feet. It also starts in the hospital, where they give you leg strengthening exercises, have you lift weights with your legs, walk the treadmill, push your leg against pressure from the therapist, etc. The goal is to try to get you to walk, first with the therapist's help, then with a cane, and finally on your own. They don't usually achieve this goal while you're in the hospital. At least they didn't with me, but my stroke was quite a serious one.

After I went home I had a visiting physical therapist and he, contrary to the first visiting occupational therapist, was excellent. I feel his work with me was very beneficial. This was not just because of what he did but what he taught me to do for myself. When he worked with me Barbara made notes of his exercises. I still use them and find them valuable over two years later. You may want to incorporate some of these in your own exercise program.

Physical Therapy Exercises

As you do these exercises, work from the bottom (feet) up.

Ankle Exercise

Lying on the bed, point your toes to ceiling and then point them forward. Keep your knees down and flat on the bed. Do 10 times on each leg. As you do the exercise, visualize the movement to reeducate the brain cells. *Any exercise you do on the right side you should also do on the left side to keep balanced.*

Heel Sliding on Bed

1. As you slide the heel back, bend your knee as much as possible. Hold it for a moment. Then, in a controlled, smooth movement, push your heel forward until you have flattened your leg. Repeat 10 times.

2. Keeping your knees close together, draw your ankles toward your bottom. Slide back and forth. Rest when you're tired; don't overdo it thinking you'll build endurance that way. Repeat 10 times.

Slide Leg Out to Side and Back

1. Lying on your bed, keep your leg flat. Slide your leg out to the side, then back to its starting position. Do it slowly. When you move the leg, do not position it at 90 degrees; try for about 45 degrees. Repeat 10 times. Do this exercise with the other leg.

2. Begin with both legs together and flat on the bed. Slide your heels out and back, like the bottom half of a jumping jack. Repeat 10 times.

Pelvic Exercises

1. Squeeze buttocks together, then relax. (This promotes pelvis stability.)

2. Bend knees. Then hold together. Roll slowly from side to side. (This improves coordination and pelvic movement.)

Bridge

Lying on your back on the bed, lift yourself up with your feet and legs, forming a "bridge" (raise your buttocks but keep your shoulder blades resting on the bed for support). Lift up and down 5 times. Rest. Do another 5 repetitions.

Rolling in Bed

A very important exercise that uses a lot of muscles. On your back, roll from side to side. Repeat 5 times on each side.

Cane Walking

This will develop balance and rhythm in your walking. Hold the cane in your left hand and place it on the ground a little forward and to your left. With your weight on your left foot, step forward on your right foot. Shift your weight onto your right foot. With your weight on the right foot, bring the left foot up beside it. Do the whole thing over and over again: Cane-Right Foot-Left Foot; Cane-Right Foot-Left Foot; Cane-Right Foot-Left Foot; Cane-Right Foot-Left Foot; Cane-Right Foot-Left Foot. When turning, always turn on your left side toward the cane. (If your stroke was on the left side, reverse this exercise.)

Miscellaneous Physical Therapy Notes
Sitting

When attempting to sit down on a chair, lean forward, then go backward. Reach back with your strong hand, touch the front edge of the seat of the chair (so you'll know where it is), and sit. Always lead with the hand.

Walking

When walking, always turn on the left side toward the cane. (If the left side is the stroke side, turn on the right side toward the cane.) Move slowly until you're more sure of yourself. If you have trouble with balancing, use a quad (four-legged) cane.

Outpatient Occupational Therapy

The first thing my occupational therapist did for me was to put a wet hot pack on my shoulder to loosen things up and improve my subluxation. After the muscles were sufficiently relaxed, she gave me many exercises. I sat at a table and moved cups back and forth. She also asked me to move balls around, sometimes having me bat at them with my stroke hand. This resulted in a noticeable improvement in the mobility of my arm. And she did get a lot of mobility back in my arm at least after the first stroke. When my regular therapist left after a month, she was replaced by a young therapist who wasn't quite as good. This was her first hospital assignment, and she seemed to be learning on the job. She didn't learn much on me, though, because after only one session, I had my second stroke. I heard that when she heard about it, she was terribly worried, thinking that something she had done had caused it. I called to reassure her that it was not her fault since I didn't want to ruin her career almost before it started.

Outpatient Physical Therapy

The physical therapist's job is to strengthen your walking, improve your balance, and build up the strength of your limbs. In my case, PT mainly involved the leg and the foot. PT is extremely important because it reminds you that you're still a functioning human being. I especially benefited from my outpatient physical therapy because I had an outstanding trainer. He helped me to strengthen my affected leg by holding it and telling me to lift it. He then would use what seemed like all his strength to not let me lift it so I had to use as much force as possible to lift it and thereby strengthen my muscles.

Then he would work on balance, maybe even having me bounce up and down on a trampoline. He helped me regain a great deal of balance and he taught me how to walk again using a long runway with bars on both sides. He would have me walk forward and backward and would always be there to support me, so I felt extremely safe. Then he got to walking me down the hospital hall. Each week he would make me walk a little farther and would keep track of how far I went. When I got weary he instantly knew it and would say, "Well, I think you've had enough for today." I really appreciated that because he listened to my body—and he listened to me. He always asked me, "Do you think you've had enough now?" But he wouldn't terminate me too early either, unless he thought I was too weak to continue.

When I returned home after the second stroke I didn't recoup so fast. I had a different home occupational therapist than the last one. She was very nice and always on time, which is something of a miracle in itself. She presented me with a set of exercises using a walker and tried to straighten out my right arm, which had a lot of spasticity—meaning it was rigidly bent at the elbow and the hand was flopped over at the wrist and clutched to my chest with my fingers making a fist. I kept doing the same exercises every week but I made so little progress that it was disheartening. Finally I gave up the visiting home therapists. It was not that they were all that different from the hospital therapists; what was all that different was me. That second stroke had pretty much broken my gung-ho spirit.

Pretty much, but not totally. What I did was use Deding, who came here every day for six hours, to help me with my therapies. We put my arm in a padded brace, which straightened out my wrist and held it down with straps. My hand eventually began opening up after I started taking Zanaflex (a muscle-relaxing medication recommended by a neurologist). That helped me a great deal psychologically as well as physically. I keep working hard at both OT and PT because *you must keep at it.* If you don't keep at it all hope is lost.

Speech Therapy

Two common effects of a stroke are dysarthia and aphasia, and they can be among the most frustrating disabilities a strokee is faced with during rehabilitation. Happily, there are many eager professionals ready to help you reclaim language.[2]

---

[2]Incidentally—or not so incidentally—speech therapists not only treat stroke-induced aphasia, but equally, if not more importantly, they help with swallowing. The therapy that is good for speech is also beneficial for swallowing because the same throat and tongue muscles control both. When I had my seizure, the person who did my swallowing test to see if I could avoid having a feeding tube inserted was a speech therapist.

Dysarthia

Dysarthia is a condition in which the strokee is no longer able to produce speech properly, due to paralysis or muscle weakness in the face and jaw muscles. Their speech may range from just slightly garbled or distorted to completely unintelligible. Strokees who face this problem also often have difficulty swallowing or chewing food as well (see "Don't Dis Dysphagia," page 109).

Aphasia

Aphasia, on the other hand, affects a strokee's ability to process language—that is, to comprehend what others are saying. Sometimes speech will sound like so many mangled words, and English will sound like a foreign language. Sometimes aphasia also affects a person's ability to comprehend the written word, as well. This can be particularly devastating. But there are many therapies available to victims of aphasia, so never fear!

Mouth Resuscitation

I had some speech therapy when I was in the hospital after my first stroke, but I discontinued it when I was discharged. My speech isn't all that bad except when I'm tired and then I chew and garble my words (unfortunately speech therapy won't drive away fatigue). At home, I still occasionally try a few of the exercises the hospital therapist taught me, lest I regress back into garble. Barbara, who has to listen to me and try to decipher when the words don't come out with crystal clarity, keeps urging me to have more speech therapy. Of course she's always urging me to have more of any and all therapies. That's the way caregivers tend to be—and strokees, who have to struggle through the therapies—tend to resist.

When Barbara was but a tot in the Midwest, it was all the vogue for children to take elocution lessons. The teacher always gave the class a warm-up exercise that Barbara keeps trying to get me to adopt. It is:

Ahh, Ooo, Eee, Ooo, I am a funny little clown.
I open my mouth wide when I say ahh.
I make my lips very round when I say ooo.
I put my teeth together when I say eee.
Ahh, Ooo, Eee, Ooo, I am a funny little clown.

Actually it's not a bad exercise—except you feel like an idiot doing it!

A far better and less ludicrous choice would be the twenty-one oral exercises created by Kathleen R. Helfrich-Miller, Ph.D., CCC, a Pittsburgh speech-language pathologist. These were originally intended for M.S. patients, but are of equal value as post-stroke therapy.

Dr. Helfrich-Miller advises you to use a mirror to help you do these exercises. Practice two to three times a day for about ten to twenty minutes. Try them all.[3]

1. Open and close your mouth slowly several times. Be sure your lips are closed all the way.
2. Pucker your lips, as for a kiss, hold, then relax. Repeat several times.
3. Spread your lips into a big smile, hold, then relax. Repeat several times.
4. Pucker, hold, smile, hold. Repeat this alternating movement several times.
5. Open your mouth, then try to pucker with your mouth

[3]Reprinted by permission of Kathleen R. Helfrich-Miller, Ph.D., CCC. Rehabilitation Specialists, Inc., 35 North Balph Avenue, Pittsburgh, PA 15202-3200; Phone: (412) 761-6062; Fax: (412) 761-7336.

wide open. Don't close your jaw. Hold, relax, and repeat several times.

6. Close your lips tightly and press together. Relax and repeat.

7. Close your lips firmly, slurp all the saliva onto the top of your tongue.

8. Open your mouth and stick out your tongue. Be sure your tongue comes straight out of your mouth and doesn't go off to the side. Hold, relax, and repeat several times. Work toward sticking your tongue out farther each day, but still pointing straight ahead.

9. Stick out your tongue and move it slowly from corner to corner of your lips. Hold in each corner, relax, and repeat several times. Be sure your tongue actually touches each corner each time.

10. Stick out your tongue and try to reach your chin with the tongue tip. Hold at the farthest point. Relax. Repeat

11. Stick out your tongue and try to reach your nose with the tongue tip. Pretend you are licking a Popsicle or cleaning some jelly from your top lip. Don't use your bottom lip or your fingers as helpers. Hold as far up as you can reach. Relax. Repeat.

12. Use a tongue depressor or spoon. Stick out your tongue. Hold the spoon against the tip of your tongue and try to push the spoon even farther away with your tongue while your hand is holding the spoon steadily in place. Hold the spoon like a Popsicle or sucker—upright, not in your mouth. Relax. Repeat.

13. Stick out your tongue. Pretend to lick a sucker, moving the tongue tip from down toward your chin to up toward your nose. Go slowly and use as much movement as you can. Relax. Repeat.

14. Stick your tongue out and pull it back, then repeat as many times as you can and as quickly as you can. Rest. Repeat.

15. Move your tongue from corner to corner as quickly as you can. Rest. Repeat.

16. Move your tongue all around your lips in a circle as quickly, but as completely, as you can, touching all of both your upper lip, corner, lower lip, and corner in your circle. Rest. Repeat.

17. Open and close your mouth as quickly as you can. Be sure your lips close each time. Rest. Repeat.

18. Say "Ma-ma-ma-ma" as quickly as you can without losing the ma sound. Be sure there's an M and an AH each time. Rest. Repeat

19. Say "La-la-la-la" as quickly and accurately as you can. Rest. Repeat.

20. Say "Ka-ka-ka-ka" as quickly as you can. Rest. Repeat.

21. Say "Kala-kala-kala-kala" as quickly and as accurately as you can. Rest. Repeat.

You can see speech therapy in action if you rent the movie *Diamonds* with Kirk Douglas. It's entertaining and very authentic since Douglas had a stroke that affected his speech, as did his character in the film. Obviously he knows—and believes in—speech therapy, since throughout the movie he keeps doing his exercises. At the end he even gets Lauren Bacall to join in with him. Watch him carefully and you can pick up some good pointers. (He does a lot of sticking out of his tongue—a basic speech therapy exercise as you can see from above.) You can see Kirk Douglas in another post-stroke film: *It Runs in the Family,* which does, indeed, feature family members, including a former wife.

If you are embarrassed by any speech problem you may have, Kirk should be an inspiration to you to get over it as he unashamedly and with verve steps up and does his acting thing. (See the write-up of Kirk Douglas's stroke in "Other People's Strokes," page 201.)

Aphasia Loves Company

Another way to prevail over feelings of chagrin and frustration and isolation is to join a support group. You can probably find one from a stroke association, hospital outpatient therapy program, speech therapist, or your physician. As Nancy A. Melville reports in her www.HealingWell.com article, "Stroke Victims Find Voice in Group Therapy; Research show supportive group setting speeds up speech improvement," ". . . group treatment offers psycho-social benefits that are just enormous because you have these people finally coming out of their homes or one-on-one therapy, and they're finding other people who are going through the very things they're going through and it's a very powerful experience for them to realize it's not such a rare thing . . . They share not only support for one another, but they wind up helping one another to benefit in communication skills as well."

Software for a Hard Problem

If you have access to a computer, you should investigate the speech software by Bungalow. This multifaceted program was developed by a speech pathologist, Terri Nichols, and her computer programmer, Clay. Their home therapy goal was that of "providing economical, high-quality software to assist in speech language recovery." Check it out at www.bungalowsoftware.com. You can even download a free trial CD or request a free floppy demo disk. Phone: 1-540-951-0623; Fax: 1-508-526-0305; e-mail: info@Bungalowsoftware.com; Mail: Bungalow Software, 2905 Wakefield Dr., Blacksburg, VA 24060-8184.

Chew, Chew, Chew, Baby

After I had been taken off the feeding tube in the hospital, I was having trouble chewing and swallowing. When Gertrude, the nurse who took care of Barbara's father after his stroke, visited me,

I complained about this. She advised me to chew gum to exercise the mouth and to get it back in action again. I did and still do this, especially since learning about the development of a new medicated xylitol gum, which I now use. As a diabetic I had always known about the sugarfree sweetener xylitol, but I didn't realize that it also removes plaque, prevents cavities, and stimulates saliva. Not only does saliva have antibiotic properties but it also helps wash away food particles that can lead to mouth infections as well as bacteria and yeast infections elsewhere in the body. This kind of gum would have obvious benefits to someone after a stroke, when their dental hygiene may not be as meticulous as before. You can order xylitol gum by phone from Homestead Market (1-800-234-1906). The flavors available are: Fresh Fruit, Spearmint, and Peppermint. As of this writing, a container of 100 pieces costs $9.95 plus shipping and handling. If you're a truly dedicated chomper, you can get 600 pieces for $47.95 plus shipping and handling.

COMPLEMENTARY AND ALTERNATIVE THERAPIES

A complementary stroke therapy is one you use in conjunction with conventional therapies. An alternative therapy is one you use *instead of* the conventional therapies. Even if you grow discouraged with the results of your standard therapies, you should never throw them all overboard and launch solely into experimentation with something newer and as yet unproved scientifically and clinically. On the other hand, in consultation with your stroke health care professionals, it's worth a try to see if one of the alternative therapies can improve your mobility and/or relieve you from pain. Many accepted theories and therapies used today started out as unproven—and even maligned—alternatives. Ignaz Phillip Semmelweis, the Hungarian obstetrician practicing in Vienna in the mid-1840s, was understandably distressed about the number of women (13 percent!) who, after giving birth, died of puerperal fever. He ultimately discovered the problem was that physicians didn't wash their hands before delivery. The simple expediency of hand washing cut the mortality rate in his hospital to 2 percent. A harmless enough practice it seemed, yet Semmelweis was so excoriated by his fellow physicians, who resented his criticism and his attempts to change their hallowed procedures, that he was ultimately driven mad.

So don't drive the alternative therapists to asylums. You never know when there's another Semmelweis out there coming up with a stroke therapy that will make a huge difference in your life and the lives of other strokees. I plan to keep looking—and so should you. Below are a few alternative and complementary therapies that might be worth a try.

Water Therapy

Water therapy is an alternative that has definitely moved into the mainstream. If you're lucky enough to have a water therapy facility in your neighborhood, this type of therapy could be beneficial for you. Water is denser than air—the muscles must work about twelve times harder in water than outside the pool—so it's possible to build more strength this way. It also doesn't feel quite as strenuous, and the cool water is comforting. Other benefits of water therapy include improved flexibility of the joints, increased stability, and even some pain reduction. Check your local yellow pages for rehabilitation centers that provide this kind of therapy. You could also find a quiet corner of your community pool and do some gentle exercises with a partner (be certain to have a buddy with you at all times in case of falls).

Water therapy provides an opportunity to move your arms and legs safely—although for some strokees, getting into that swimsuit can prove tricky. All in all, it's a very soothing technique. If you can handle the logistics of the situation (finding a driver, a good water therapist, and a tangle-free swimsuit), you might want to give it a try.

Craniosacral Therapy—Soft Touch

The basic theory of craniosacral therapy is that a fluid called cerebro-spinal fluid (CSF) is produced in the brain and rhythmically pumped throughout the head and spine. In treatment, the patient—fully clothed—lies on a massage table. A trained therapist, using gentle touching—mainly on the head, with pressure no heavier than the weight of a quarter—evaluates the different parts of the body and determines if there is a blockage of the flow of CSF, which one practitioner calls "the moving tide of life." Blockages, so the theory goes, cause the rhythm of the body to be disrupted. The practitioner then treats the blockages with a gentle touching to open the flow and improve the functioning of the central nervous system.

The therapist often has a helper or helpers in the session. Deding was taught to help me during mine by holding one part of my leg. Barbara was told to hold another part and sometimes there were other helpers who encouraged the cerebro-spinal fluid to move the way it should through targeted touching.

Craniosacral therapy was originated by Dr. John Upledger, an osteopathic physician and a professor of biomechanics at Michigan State University. He developed his theory after assisting a neurosurgeon's operation and observing the pulsing of the cerebro-spinal fluid. This led him to discover techniques to improve the action of the cerebro-spinal fluid and thereby improve the various health problems of his patients.

At this time, unfortunately, few health insurance plans/companies pay for this particular therapy, and it can cost about $100 an hour. I only had five sessions before deciding that craniosacral therapy didn't seem to be helping me. The therapist wanted me to continue therapy for about a year, but I couldn't see tying up that much of my life—and money!—lying on a table with the therapist touching my head. But maybe you'll have better luck. It's possible that I gave it up too soon. I'm an impatient person. There are many true believers in craniosacral therapy who cite amazing results in children with learning disabilities as well as people with high blood pressure and chronic pain and allergies.

You may want to give it a try and assess it for yourself. One thing I will say about craniosacral therapy though, from even my limited experience: it is by far the easiest, most pleasant therapy I've ever experienced—just lying there with people gently touching you. It's a far cry from the hard work most therapies require, and that relaxation may be worth the price of admission.[4]

Constraint-Induced Movement Therapy

Still in its experimental phase, there is a hopeful new development on the stroke therapy scene: constraint-induced movement therapy (CIM), also known as forced use therapy. The way this works is that the strong arm is bandaged and tied down, rendered as immobile as if it were bound in a mummy's wrap. The stroke-damaged arm then must be used to complete everyday tasks. (You could compare it to learning to write with your left hand if you've broken your right—but with the whole arm rendered useless rather than just the hand.) The goal of CIM therapy is for the patient to use their affected side for 90 percent of their waking hours, keeping the other arm under constraint.

---

[4] To find out more about craniosacral therapy you can contact The Upledger Institute, Inc., 11211 Prosperity Farms Road, Suite D-325, Palm Beach Gardens, FL 33410; Phone: 561-622-4706; Fax: 561-622-4771; e-mail: upledger@upledger.com. There are also many references and articles on cranial-sacral therapy on the Internet.

Dr. Edward Taub, a neuroscientist at the University of Alabama, maintains that a number of cells are killed outright in a stroke, but other cells surrounding the injury are only stunned. The theory is that CIM therapy with the stroke arm can reorganize the brain and wake up some "stunned" cells, resulting in improved arm use. Dr. Taub reports that more than 150 stroke patients have been treated with CIM therapy at the University of Alabama and at the Friedrich-Schiller University in Germany. All have improved mobility, some regaining a great deal of movement. And so far, the improvements seem to be permanent.

This is not an easy therapy. Those involved with CIM are expected to work six or seven hours a day for two to three weeks. This is more than many patients can handle, especially those who are elderly.

The other not-so-great news is that the cost of the program for a patient at university treatment centers can range from $6,000 to $13,000, not covered by Medicare or private insurance. At the University of Alabama, only five new patients start the program each week, and there are five thousand on the waiting list. But there are other clinics that offer this kind of therapy.

Even if you can't handle a CIM program either physically or financially, there is one thing you can learn from it. As Dr. Taub points out, "Right after a stroke, a limb is paralyzed. Whenever the person tries to move an arm, it simply doesn't work. Even when the cells that represent the arm in the brain are not dead, the patient, expecting failure, stops trying to use it. We call this learned non-use."[5]

Keep that in mind and make a conscious effort to keep trying to use the so-called "bad arm" or "bad hand" every day. You could

[5] Drug Resource Center. "Pushing Injured Brains and Spinal Cords to New Paths," August 28, 2001, Birmingham, Ala. (*New York Times* News Service).

even go so far as to keep the hand of the good arm in your pocket or the thumb hooked on your belt so it won't try to get into the act. Just pretend that the stroke arm and hand are all you have to use and see if slowly, gradually over time your "let's pretend therapy" may start to induce a little movement in the formerly paralyzed hand and arm . . . and then a little more, until who knows what might happen, as long as you keep those two New York Public Library Lions, Patience and Fortitude, on the job!

Stroke Recovery Systems' NeuroMove

When I went back to the rehab facility for a tune-up, I became acquainted with a next-room neighbor with whom I had diabetes in common. When he heard about my stroke he told me about the experience of a friend's mother-in-law. Three years previously she had a stroke, which left her with a severely hemiplegic right arm and hand. Through her husband, who is a retired physician, she heard about Stroke Recovery Systems' NeuroMove. The NeuroMove, which has been approved by the FDA specifically for stroke rehab, is only about the size of a clock radio and can be easily stored and used at home. It is comprised of three sensors and the NeuroMove itself, which contains a computer and has a display screen.

This woman obtained one and, after working with it regularly for several months, was able to perform such feats as raising her arm above her head and—most amazing of all for this avid bridge player—to shuffle cards. She called the NeuroMove "a miracle."

Basically, what's going on in this kind of therapy is biofeedback. Put simply, this means learning to control your bodily functions with the power of your mind. To give you an idea of how biofeedback works, think of a lemon and see if it makes your mouth water. You can also learn to warm your hands by simply concentrating on your hands growing warmer and warmer and warmer. Conversely, if you find yourself sweating in the heat of summer, your air conditioner conked out, and you think of cold substances, like ice, glaciers—even Antarctica!—you may discover that you feel significantly cooler.

Once you've proven to yourself that you can make your mouth water and your hands grow warm through the power of your mind, it's not that much of a stretch to convince yourself that you can also make dormant neurons and muscles wake up and live.

The way the NeuroMove works is that its three sensors are attached to the skin above muscle groups that you want to bring back to life. You then concentrate on moving those muscles. When the NeuroMove detects any activity in that area—no matter how minute and invisible—the unit "rewards" you with a few seconds of muscle contraction. This is an important element in relearning the movement, and those who have used the Neuro-Move say it's very motivating to feel those muscles, which have been nearly paralyzed since the stroke, contract. It gives them hope. Most patients use the NeuroMove up to three times a day for twenty-minute periods.

Admittedly, there are, the company explains, certain situations in which NeuroMove will not work: when a patient is not cognitively intact (author's translation: has dementia), is confused, not able to concentrate on simple tasks, or is simply unmotivated. The NeuroMove requires a physician's prescription.[6]

Botox: Both a Therapy and a Medication

There are no magic elixirs to bring you back to normal functioning instantly. There is only hard work on self-rehabilitation . . .

---

[6] For further information, including cost and lease options, contact www.neuromove.com or Stroke Recovery Systems, 8100 South Park Way, #A1, Littleton, CO 80120; Phone: (800) 845-1771 or (303) 707-0203; Fax: (800) 495-6695 or (303) 347-9153; Internet: www. neuromove.com.

and time, lots of time. That being the case, think how excited we were then when we first heard about Botox for relaxation of the muscles of the elbow and wrist so you don't have to suffer the classic stroke position of the arm rigidly bent at the elbow held next to your chest and the wrist (again rigidly) bent downward. We were hopeful that maybe there would even be a return to some usefulness for eating, writing, and so on.

This is the same Botox, the benign poison that people use successfully, albeit temporarily, to remove wrinkles, especially on the forehead and lines around the mouth. The downsides to Botox are a somewhat painful injection with a mega-syringe by a physician and its expense: around $400 to $600 a pop. On average, a Botox injection lasts approximately three months. This treatment may or may not be covered by insurance, but at least you will have a better chance of having the procedure covered than those using the injections to remove wrinkles, since in your case, it would be a therapeutic procedure, not cosmetic.

Barbara was ecstatic when she learned about Botox. She was certain this was what we had been waiting for—the perfect quick-fix that would make things the way they used to be, including our lives. She actually had the totally unrealistic idea that after one shot I would suddenly regain total use of my right hand and arm and would be able to play tennis or the violin with it—if I knew how to play either tennis or the violin, that is.

I, on the other hand, was more skeptical. I had read a study by the company that produces Botox that it was shown to have worked on 60 percent of strokees, but not on the other 40 percent. Was I going to be part of the happy 60 percent or one of the dejected 40 percent? All I could do was try and see.

My highly competent and incredibly conscientious physical medicine and rehabilitation doctor started off slowly, trying a low dosage shot for my bent wrist and warning that it would take a week or two before I saw results. She also advised me to get an orthotic brace for my right arm and hand. I was to wear this several hours a day; she would then increase the force of the brace to straighten the arm enough so that another Botox injection could be given—this time in the arm. This would, we hoped, drop the arm enough to return some of its normal function. (If I used the orthotic alone, it would take up to a year to straighten the arm. With the orthotic *and* Botox, it should take only six to eight weeks.)

Despite Barbara's relentless nagging, I delayed getting the orthotic. After two years I was mightily sick of going to doctors and therapists and getting a succession of special devices—usually to no avail—and I wanted to see if the Botox alone would work. It didn't. So, I reluctantly went to the orthotic service, where the therapist fitted the brace to my arm, warning that if I had too much pain or redness under the apparatus, I should immediately discontinue using it. For me, the pain was so excruciating that after two and a half hours, I had Deding remove it. Red spots were already developing on the skin.

Barbara was heartbroken, the doctor was disappointed, the elbow and wrist were as rigidly locked as ever, but I was out of pain and at peace. The odds didn't work for me on this one, but you may be in the Botox blesséd 60 percent, so it is worth a try. I wish you well!

MEDICATIONS

As you must have noticed, strokees often have a medicine cabinet full of medications—some related to stroke-related problems (maladies that resulted from the stroke) and others to prevent future strokes.

We won't go into detail about the medications (this is something you should discuss with your physician). Instead, we'll provide a brief overview of some of the most common stroke-related medications. This doesn't mean you shouldn't learn all you can about the medications you take! And besides your doctor, an excellent source of valuable information regarding medicines is your pharmacist. He or she can not only explain the pertinent facts of a medication to you, but can make sure it won't cause an adverse reaction with other medications you may be taking. In addition, your pharmacist is far more accessible than your doctor—no appointments necessary! To make life easier, you should obtain all of your medications from the same pharmacy. Your medical history and your prescription information will be on file, making it easier for the pharmacist to check on you when you come in with a new prescription or have questions about an existing medicine you are taking.

Blood Thinners, Anti-Clotting Medicines, and Cholesterol-Lowering Drugs

Aspirin

Aspirin is an antiplatelet that decreases blood clot formation by keeping the smallest blood cells (platelets) from sticking together to form clots. Aspirin is the most popular stroke-preventing medication, and the most accessible. Regular use (consult your doctor or pharmacist for appropriate dosage) reduces the chance of stroke in people who have already suffered a TIA or stroke, as well as people who have significant hardening or narrowing of arteries, particularly the carotid, which can lead to heart attack, stroke, and peripheral vascular disease.

Clopidogrel (brand name Plavix)

Clopidogrel is another antiplatelet, commonly used to prevent and treat heart attack, stroke, blood clots, and acute coronary syndrome.

Dipyridamole (brand name Persantine)
Dipyridamole prevents platelets from sticking together or attaching to prosthetic heart valve surfaces. It is often used to prevent blood clots that form after heart surgery.

Lovastatin (brand names Altocor, Mevacor)
Lovastatin blocks the production of cholesterol, reduces total cholesterol and LDL (or "bad") cholesterol.

Pravastatin (brand name Pravachol)
Pravastatin blocks the production of cholesterol, reduces total cholesterol, LDL cholesterol, triglycerides, and apolipoprotein B (a protein that makes cholesterol).

Simvastatin (brand name Zocor)
Like pravastatin, simvastatin blocks the production of cholesterol, reduces total cholesterol, LDL cholesterol, triglycerides, and apolipoprotein B. It also increases HDL (or "good") cholesterol.

Ticlopidine (brand name Ticlid)
Ticlopidine prevents blood platelets from clustering and forming clots. It is used to prevent strokes in patients who have already suffered a TIA or stroke.

Warfarin (brand name Coumadin)
Warfarin is an anticoagulant, or blood thinner, that reduces the formation of blood clots. It is an important tool in the prevention of heart attacks, vein and artery blockage, and further strokes. Vitamin K, found mainly in liver and green, leafy vegetables like broccoli, Brussels sprouts, collards, and cabbage, decreases the drug's effectiveness. Your doctor will likely warn you off such foods while you are on Coumadin.

BLOOD PRESSURE–LOWERING MEDICATIONS (ANTIHYPERTENSIVES)

High blood pressure is an extreme stroke risk. If making the appropriate lifestyle adjustments (losing weight, exercising, cutting back on salt, cutting out or limiting alcohol) doesn't bring down your blood pressure, you will need the help of a blood pressure–lowering medication. Sometimes it takes a combination of medications to get the desired effect. Since everyone is different and reacts differently to these medications, there is no concrete formula. Your doctor may have to try different medicines to see what works best for you. When he or she finds the medication that brings your blood pressure into the correct range, that's good news—but the news isn't so good that you can stop taking the medication! Stroke medications are often something that will be a reality for the rest of your life, although sometimes the dosage can be lowered.

There are four major categories of blood pressure medications: diuretics, beta-blockers, ACE inhibitors, ARBs angiostensin II receptors.

Diuretics

Because diuretics are effective and inexpensive, they are often the first drug people turn to for blood pressure management. Commonly called "water pills" because they increase the frequency of urination, diuretics cause kidneys to eliminate sodium and water, which relaxes the blood vessel walls, thereby lowering blood pressure. They are frequently combined with other antihypertensive medications to enhance their effectiveness. Diuretics are especially beneficial for older adults and the overweight.

Beta-Blockers

Beta-blockers are medications that reduce blood pressure by decreasing both the heart rate and the amount of blood the heart pumps out with each beat. These can be used alone or in combination with a diuretic.

ACE Inhibitors

Angiotensin-converting enzyme (ACE) inhibitors reduce blood pressure by blocking the enzyme that narrows blood vessels, making it easier for the blood to flow through. The drug further lowers blood pressure by increasing the release of water and sodium in the urine. ACE inhibitors can be used alone or combined with a diuretic or other antihypertensive.

Angiotensin II Receptor Blockers

These drugs also block the action of a hormone that causes blood vessels to narrow, consequently causing blood vessels to relax and widen. This makes it easier for blood to flow through the vessels, which reduces blood pressure. They can be used alone or with other antihypertensives.

GENERIC DRUGS

During recovery I had an adventure with my blood pressure. Using 50 milligrams of Zestril (an ACE inhibitor) per day I always kept my blood pressure in the 120 to 130 range. If it sneaked over the upper border, I had permission from my doctor to add another 10 milligrams. I take my blood pressure every day so I can spring into action if it goes higher than it should be.

This particular morning I was aghast to see that my blood pressure had soared to 170. Maybe it was a mistake, I thought, an

operator error. took my blood pressure again an hour later, and
there was no change. I took the 10 extra milligrams of Zestril generic I had been using, and a couple of hours later it was 179!

Barbara and I started pondering if anything had changed in
my therapy or my life that might have caused this sudden rise in
blood pressure. We couldn't think of anything—but someone else
could. Dedirg, my other—and obviously more perspicacious!—
caregiver pointed out that my blood pressure had started going up
when I changed—for cost considerations—to the generic version
of Zestril. When she checked with her sister (a nurse), the sister
said that I definitely shouldn't abruptly change to a generic because my system had grown accustomed to the brand name. The
generic could cause problems with my therapy.

Luckily, I still had some 10-milligram tablets of the "real thing"
on hand and shifted back to that. The next morning my blood
pressure was 114 and it has continued in the good old familiar
range ever since. Of course, in a recent cost-cutting spasm, my
health insurance now charges a $15 co-pay for the non-generic as
opposed to a $5 co-pay for the generic, but it's worth it for nor-
mal blood pressure. This is not to say that generic drugs do not
work as effectively as brand names; most do. However, there are
times when the "real thing" is worth the extra cost. Your health,
as they say, is priceless.

Is It All Right to Use Generic Drugs?

Before we answer that, we'd like you to have an understanding of
what generic drugs are. Barbara and I had long been confused
about them ourselves, so we asked the pharmacist of a company
with which we were once affiliated to explain them. The first thing
we discovered surprised us: Pharmacies actually make a greater
percentage of profit on generics than on brand names, so if your
pharmacist discourages you from purchasing a certain generic in

favor of the brand name, he's doing it for professional reasons and not out of some sordid profit motive. Conversely, this shouldn't lead you to believe that should a pharmacist suggest a generic, he or she is not being straight with you. It's important to cultivate a trusting relationship with your neighborhood pharmacist to avoid misunderstandings and sticky situations that might crop up.

Our pharmacist friend further explained that generic drugs (drugs not protected by trademark) are in demand today for many valid reasons. First, insurance companies and other health-cost payment systems are encouraging their members to use generic drugs by offering them a lower co-payment. (The pharmacy we use has posted this sign: "Due to mandatory generic substitutions on most insurance plans, your doctor must *physically indicate* 'Do not substitute' on the prescription to receive a brand-name medication.") Second, the FDA is shortening the time period for trade-name drugs to become generic. And thirdly, over the next three to four years, if the federal government (Medicare) phases in payments for prescription drugs (just as the state of California now does with its Medi-Cal drug program), it will probably demand that generic medications be provided whenever possible.

With the following classes of drugs, you, your doctor, and pharmacist must be extremely careful when changing to the generic form.

- cardiovascular drugs (digoxin, Inderal, etc.)
- hormone and related drugs (Premarin)
- psychotherapeutic drugs (Thorazine, Elavil, etc.)
- anticonvulsants (Dilantin)
- oral hypoglycemics (Orinase, Diabenese, etc.)

For the above reasons, it's safe to say that generics are here to stay. But buyer beware! Some warnings are in order. Brand-name drugs and their generic forms are not necessarily identical. Switching to a generic without proper precautions may cause serious problems (like mine). To understand the possible difficulties, you have to understand what generic drugs are and how they're made.

A generic drug has exactly the same amount of the active ingredient as the trade-name product. The active ingredient by weight, however, makes up only a fraction of the total weight of the tablet or capsule. For example, a Lanoxin 0.25 milligram tablet weighs about 1.5 milligrams, but the active ingredient (digoxin) makes up only about 10 percent of the total weight of the tablet. The other 90 percent comprises what pharmacists call excipients—fillers, binding agents, coloring, etc. It is these extra ingredients that very often determine how much of the active drug is absorbed into the bloodstream and how quickly. In some cases more drug is absorbed and in other cases less. This difference can be critical, depending on the type of drug you're using.

Before switching (or being switched!) to a generic you should check with your doctor, as I didn't. It's just fortunate that I have my own blood pressure monitor at home and am so diligent about checking it or I might have run this high blood pressure until it was discovered in my next visit to the doctor with who knows what dire results. I would advise any person who has had a stroke or even a TIA to invest in a home blood pressure monitor and use it regularly. Incidentally, if you use a home blood pressure monitor, it's important that you position your arm carefully and correctly. A study from the University of California, San Diego, concluded that with the arm straight and parallel to the body you can get a reading that is up to 10 percent higher than if the elbow is bent at a right angle to the body at the level of the heart. The ideal position, they say, is with the arm at heart level and the elbow just slightly flexed.

The final word on generics, then, is to go ahead and enjoy the savings they offer, but make sure that you, your physician, and your pharmacist work as a team to ensure their safe and efficacious use.

EMERGENCY MEASURES

Clot-Busters and Bat Spit to the Rescue

It is axiomatic that it's vitally important to take emergency measures as quickly as possible after a stroke because "time is brain." The longer you delay the more likely it is that the brain will be damaged—often irreparably so. Currently there is only one drug (rt-PA) approved by the FDA to treat acute ischemic strokes. The problem with this drug is that to be safe and effective it must be administered within the first three hours after the stroke. This is hardly enough time to recognize that there's something wrong, and get the strokee to the hospital where they can run tests to analyze the situation and start treatment.

Fortunately there are some new developments on the stroke treatment scene that may soon become standard emergency procedures and thereby save lives and reduce stroke damage.

Clot-Busters X 2

Studies and research at the UCLA Medical Center are giving help and hope for nipping strokes in the bud (exactly where strokes need to be nipped!) in two new ways One is a drug, the other a device.

Clot-Buster #1: Magnesium Sulfate

Magnesium sulfate (Epsom salt!), a drug with few risks or side effects, is being used in a pilot study for treating ischemic strokes. It does this both by dilating blood vessels to increase blood flow to the brain and by blocking the buildup of damaging calcium in injured nerve cells. The pilot study, "Field Administration of Stroke Therapy-Magnesium Sulfate (FAST-MAG)," is a two-fold test of both the efficacy of the drug and the importance of speed in getting it to the patient. Paramedics play an important part in the study since they are the ones to administer the drug when they arrive on the scene or on the way to the hospital. As Jeffrey Saver, M.D., professor of neurology at the David Geffen School of Medicine at UCLA and one of the investigators of the study, says, "If we're going to find a benefit from neuro-protective drugs, we need to get it to the patients early. Paramedics are uniquely positioned to accelerate conventional stroke care and deliver brain-protective drugs."

The study is being conducted in conjunction with the Los Angeles County Emergency Medical Services system with paramedics from thirty provider agencies and all paramedic receiving hospitals. In an initial pilot study (May 2000 to January 2002) in which twenty patients, after having been screened for stroke by the paramedics, were given intravenous magnesium sulfate, the results were promising with the patients showing better-than-usual recovery. Incidentally, every stroke was correctly diagnosed by the paramedics. That doesn't surprise me. In my encounters with the Los Angeles paramedics, I found them to be uniformly wonderfully knowledgeable and capable, not to mention kind and caring.

Now the study is in full gear and a May 21, 2004, Reuters Health Information article by Will Boggs, M.D., trumpets its success with the headline "Prehospital neuroprotective stroke safe and feasible." In the article, Dr. Saver also delivered the glad tidings that "Based in part on the successful results of the pilot trial, we have received a $13 million, four-year award from the National Institutes of Health to perform a pivotal phase 3 trial." Dr. Saver explained the study "will compare magnesium sulfate versus placebo among 1,298 ambulance transported patients with acute stroke, with study agent [the magnesium sulfate] initiated within two hours of onset in all patients, and within one hour of onset in half [of the patients]."

Clot-Buster #2: The MERCI Retriever

MERCI stands for mechanical embolus removal in cerebral ischemia. Still in its experimental phase, this corkscrewlike tool manually extracts clots that deprive the brain of the oxygen it needs.

"This device could save lots of lives and lessen the level of disability so people can go home rather than being institutionalized," says Marilyn Rymer, a spokesperson for the National Stroke Association in Englewood, Colorado.

This is being tested on people ineligible for the current therapy approved for stroke, the aforementioned rt-PA. Unlike rt-PA, which has to be administered within three hours of the stroke, the MERCI Retriever can be used up to eight hours. Other advantages are that it saves more brain tissue because it works much faster than the drug, which takes an hour to do the job. It can also remove larger clots that are beyond the powers of the drug to dissolve. On top of everything else, unlike the drug, which can cause cerebral hemorrhages, it can be used on patients with a propensity for bleeding.

Just how does this ingenious device work? Basically it's a thin tube containing a wire made of nickel titanium, an alloy that can change shape. The tube is inserted into a blood vessel in the groin and pushed up through the body and into the brain. When it arrives at the clot, the wire is pushed out and it promptly coils into a corkscrew that grabs the clot. The comparison is made that it works in much the same way a corkscrew does when you extract a cork from a bottle of wine. At the same time the MERCI releases a small balloon that inflates to stop blood flow and prevent a second stroke in case a scrap of the clot breaks off before it is removed. The wire is then carefully pulled, extracting the clot, to be sucked out of the body with a syringe.

Now this rendition doesn't make the process seem like an enjoyable experience. But think of the joy at the outcome of the first UCLA MERCI patient as reported by Lauren Neergard of the Associated Press (October 22, 2003).

"Dr. Sidney Starkman, co-director of the UCLA Stroke Center, recalls the first patient ever treated. Five usually staid doctors jumped up and down and high-fived as a man completely paralyzed for six hours began speaking on the operating table. 'It still brings chills to me,' Starkman says."

Consider the chills it must have brought to the patient himself when he learned of his "miracle recovery."

Bat Spit (Desmoteplase)

On the bat's back I do fly . . . merrily, merrily shall I live now.

—SHAKESPEARE, *The Tempest*

The vampire bat, a thumb-size Latin American creature, feeds on the blood of sleeping mammals. In order to extend the dinner hour, a protein in the bat's saliva keeps the blood flowing and free from clots until the bat's hunger is assuaged.

At the twenty-ninth International Stroke conference in San Diego, February 5–7, 2004, Steven Warach, M.D., Ph.D., chief of the section on stroke diagnostics and therapeutics at the National Institute of Neurological Disorders and Stroke, presented the results of his study of a new drug, desmoteplase. This genetically engineered version of the bat's saliva flings open the window of opportunity for treatment of stroke to a more doable nine hours. Dr. Warach says that early studies of desmoteplase—based on forty-three stroke patients—indicate that the drug can reverse the stroke symptoms of difficulty in speaking and paralysis in 60 percent of the patients treated with the drug.

Besides the time factor, other ways in which desmoteplase trumps rt-PA is that it can dissolve a clot in the brain without increasing the risk of bleeding in other areas of the body and brain, and it is believed that it will work in more patients (rt-PA is only effective for one in eight).

Howard Rowley of the University of Wisconsin Medical School says of Dr. Warach's study, "This is the biggest breakthough I've seen in twenty years."

Four medical centers in the United States have ordered desmoteplase and will soon be testing it in their emergency rooms. Creed Pettigrew, M.D., of the University of Kentucky College of Medicine, one of the testing centers, says of desmoteplase, "I think it will revolutionize the way acute stroke care is rendered in this country."

CONQUERING CONSTIPATION

If I'm the woman who's had everything then I'm also the woman who's tried everything to conquer constipation. You might say I'm obsessed by it. Why? Because I'm certain that it caused my first stroke. Since I've always feared a repeat performance, I've searched everywhere to find information—in books and newspaper and magazine articles and on the Internet. Now I'm passing along what I've learned to you.

The most important thing for you to learn early on is that you must take constipation extremely seriously. The doctors that oversaw my hospital stay considered my idea that constipation and concomitant straining at stool could have caused the stroke ludicrous—just another loony theory from an ignorant layperson.

But I didn't give up pursuing this idea, and the higher up I went on the medical food chain, the more substantiation I received. My gynecologist said, "Of course that could have caused it. The pressure on the blood vessels from straining at stool is tremendous. As a matter of fact, even a hearty sneeze can cause a break in a blood vessel." Virginia Valentine, the nurse practitioner with whom we collaborated on our book *Diabetes, Type 2 and What to Do*, echoed my gynecologist's sentiments:

"Yes, certainly straining at stool can cause increased intracranial and intrathoracic pressure. That's exactly why they give post-MI [myocardial infarction] patients stool softeners in the ICU. It is also why we recommend folks with diabetes don't engage in lifting heavy weights, because of the increased blood pressure when they strain to lift the weights." Another nurse, Joy Pape, an expert on the low carbohydrate diet (which sometimes causes constipation) agrees, telling me: "As for the straining, Virginia is right, and it is a basic I have been taught to teach patients."

A cardiologist friend of mine bemoaned the fact that doctors seldom, if ever, warn patients against straining at stool, despite the fact that a stroke caused by this is more common than most people realize. It can bring down anyone—even a king. A friend who was a reporter on the *Memphis Commercial Appeal* at the time Elvis Presley died, told me rumors circulated in the newsroom that a stroke caused by straining at stool was what did him in. His last words were purported to be, "I'm going to the bathroom to read." (Of course if, as some people believe, Elvis still lives, then these rumors have no validity.)

But supposing you have—or develop—a recurring constipation problem, what then? Certainly you should tell your doctor about it. He or she may prescribe a stool softener. Take it. Laxatives like Colace (or Pericolace, which has an added stool softener) and a fiber supplement such as Metamucil are often recommended by health professionals. In the case of somewhat more serious bouts of constipation, you can try glycerin suppositories. If the condition persists, you can have your caregiver, a non-squeamish relative, or *very* close friend give you an enema. Actually, if you don't have hemiplegia (paralysis on one side of the body) you can probably give one to yourself. It's not all that difficult to follow the instructions and diagram on the box.

For preventive maintenance, by all means take those good old faithful home remedies, like prunes and roughage. I now have a couple prunes for breakfast most mornings, and when I need a blood-sugar-raising snack for my diabetes, prunes it is. When fresh figs are in season they are a delicious alternative to provide the same noble result. If you serve them with yogurt, you get a double-whammy laxative effect. Actually, I got acquainted with figs and yogurt long before my stroke days; in the book *From Russia with Love,* James Bond had them for breakfast, along with Turkish coffee, when he was in Istanbul. (The laxative propen-

---

High-Fiber Foods for Maintaining Regularity

Garlic

Apples

Pineapple

Papaya (one of my favorites since my first trip to Hawaii)

Raspberries

Broccoli (not for strokees on Coumadin or any other blood thinner)

Cabbage (not for strokees on Coumadin or any other blood thinner)

Beans of all kinds (cooking them in a Crock-Pot is the easy way to go.
   See "Slow Cooker," pg. 113).

High-fiber cereals, breads, and muffins (look for the fiber content on
   the label)

sities weren't mentioned.) Pears are also good because they contain sorbitol, which has a lively laxative effect, as anyone who has ever gobbled down several pieces of sorbitol-sweetened candy can tell you.

I feel that water is a vitally important component of the anti-constipation equation. I strive valiantly to drink the requisite eight glasses of water a day, but, alas, I seldom succeed. A friend of Barbara's went to an acupuncturist, who prescribed a before-breakfast large—make that *huge*—glass of water. The man held his hands about twelve inches apart—one above the other—to indicate the size the glass should be. He told Barbara's friend that this water activates your yang (in Chinese philosophy it connotes light, air, sun, activity, brightness, etc.—the opposite of yin). Although I try to take a morning dose of what we now call "yang water," I can only manage about a third as much as the acupuncturist prescribed. I knew I couldn't handle more. Barbara's friend decided the same thing, mainly because she played in a recorder group and knew the other players wouldn't put up with the number of bathroom breaks a full measure of yang water would require.

But my most important suggestion—make that *command*—is for you to regard extreme, impacted constipation of the sort that I had as a medical emergency and to go immediately to your doctor or a proctologist and get yourself de-impacted. If it happens on a weekend—as most medical emergencies do—head straight for the emergency room. Don't let embarrassment of going there for such a "minor complaint" stop you, and don't let the personnel there fob you off and not take your condition seriously. Just flat-out state loud and clear, "I have been warned that impacted constipation of this sort can bring on a hemorrhagic stroke." Take it from one it happened to.

In his book *Happiness Is a Serious Problem,* Dennis Prager explains that Judaism has a prayer of gratitude over relieving one's body that many religious Jews always say upon leaving the bathroom. When I read this before my stroke, I thought it was a really funny thing to pray about, but now I realize that I was wrong. It is a happening truly worthy of appreciation—even veneration.

SEX AND THE STROKEE

Psychosexual therapist Dr. Ruth Westheimer, who ought to know, says that there is very little information available about sex after a stroke. That is true even when you look where you would logically expect to find it. For example, the book *My Year Off* by British editor Robert McCrum, is the story of a newly married (only two weeks!) forty-two-year-old who was struck down by a cerebral hemorrhage. His story is, as the book jacket says, "written with candor and detail," and so it is in terms of the therapies he endured and the preparations for the happy ending of the birth of his daughter; but when it came to sex, nothing. Possibly I overlooked something, but I did read the book twice. Perhaps it was a matter of British reticence, or maybe he and his wife had no problems whatsoever in their sexual relationship. In the other personal experience stroke books I read, mostly by Americans, it was much the same: a curtain of mystery was drawn across the bedroom door.

As with any and all post-stroke problems, you are always advised to check with your doctor regarding sex after a stroke. But if the truth be told, most doctors are so overworked they hardly have time to take your blood pressure, let alone engage in lengthy discussions of your sexual activities. And many of them are not comfortable giving this kind of advice, even if they had the time. Better is the advice of the formidable Dr. Ruth that when you need help with post-stroke sexual difficulties, "counseling is the best way of proceeding." And for those who cannot afford the expense of sexual therapists, she says, "If you call a teaching hospital in your area, they may have a clinic that offers counseling with fees that are on a sliding scale according to income."

Other ways you might find help in finding a therapist are by contacting social workers in local hospitals, and if there is a university nearby, you could check with their psychology department. If you do decide to go into therapy, it is important—make that *imperative*—that for a successful outcome, you and your partner must both be involved in the sessions, sometimes together and sometimes alone.

If you want to do some background reading either on your own or in conjunction with therapy, here's where our old reliable Internet comes on the scene. There you can find Web sites that can enlighten you on topics of interest on the subject of sex after a stroke.

Some important things you can learn there include:

1. This is said repeatedly: Don't worry about sexual activity bringing on a stroke. It rarely happens. Of course there's always that inevitable "check with your doctor" recommendation. But according to the Heart and Stroke Foundation of Canada, "There is no evidence that sexual activity with your usual partner can cause a heart attack or stroke. Sex is a form of physical activity that causes the heart to work harder and raises blood pressure. If you can walk up two flights of stairs with ease, your heart is probably ready for sex."

2. If you were sexually active prior to your stroke, you are more likely to be so afterward. If you had little or no interest in sex prior to your stroke, that probably won't change for the better because of the stroke.

3. The American Heart Association's Learn and Live Web site (www.justmove.org) alerts you to the fact that "Some medications, for example tranquilizers, sleeping pills, high blood

pressure medicines, antidepressants and antihistamines, can reduce sexual ability, and some can even cause impotence." If you suspect this may be a problem, don't take yourself off the drug on your own. "Never stop taking a medication without consulting your physician first."

4. Depression is the enemy of sexual intimacy, so if you have the symptoms of depression, such as lack of energy, feelings of sadness and hopelessness, sleeping too little—or too much—irritability, a negative outlook on life, etc., you should tell your doctor. This condition is treatable with antidepressants.

5. Elderly stroke patients and those with disabilities can—and do!—have active and satisfying sexual relations.

6. Keep your sense of humor alive. On the Web site www.mothernature.com/Library/Bookshelf/Books/12/21. cfm, Domeena Renshaw, M.D., director of the Sexual Dysfunction Clinic at Loyola University of Chicago Stritch School of Medicine, says, "Keep laughing. Sex at any age and with any physical problem is better if you don't take it too seriously. Have fun, be frivolous, use your imagination. Remember you're not at a stockholders' meeting—you're with someone you love. Enjoy it."

On this same Web site there is a quote that shows that a sense of humor is alive and well at the home of Jim and Cathy Kalal in Harlan, Ohio. Jim, a retired public utility administrator in his sixties, survived a paralyzing stroke in 1982. "We're keeping on pace with the national record for sex in a month by a stroke survivor," he says laughing. "I'm holding up my end."

Cathy Kalal, who is an RN, says, "I don't think you should ever give intimacy up because of a disability. You find what is the best way for you to fulfill your intimacy with each other.

We've managed to do that. We're probably as sexually active as some of the younger couples in the neighborhood."

For specific questions on stroke and sex, the Internet is invaluable. On your computer—or on any computer you can get your hands on—enter "Stroke and Sex" on a search engine (Google, Yahoo, etc.). Then you should call up and read all of the items you find there. You may discover answers to questions you didn't even think of or may have been too embarrassed to ask. Examples: different positions for those with paralysis, how to have sex when you are using a urinary catheter, choosing the best time for intercourse, other satisfying ways to be sexual with your partner, etc.

SAFETY FIRST, LAST, AND ALWAYS

Out of this nettle, danger, we pluck this flower, safety.

—SHAKESPEARE, *Henry IV*

The Harder We Fall

In the darkly humorous hospital novel *The House of God* by Samuel Shem, M.D., "Fats," the cynical resident doctor, calls particularly irritating patients—usually older ones—who repeatedly show up at the hospital "Gomers." This stands for "Get Out of My Emergency Room." He complains that "Gomers never die," meaning they'll keep coming back to the hospital emergency room, bugging the staff forever. In addition, "Fats" complains, "Gomers go to ground," meaning they're always falling.

I guess I could be categorized as a Gomer because since the beginning of my TIA and stroke days, I've been to the ER six times—surprisingly not any for falls. While it's comforting to know that I'll never die, it's discouraging to think that I'm likely to keep "going to ground." It's true that falling is one thing some of us stroke folk definitely and repeatedly do.

In his book *Cyclops Awakes; a Newspaperman Fights Back After a Massive Stroke,* John E. Mantle writes that after his stroke he fell so often that around the office his colleagues started grading his falls the way gymnasts are graded in the Olympics. I don't think I've had any falls that would earn a Nadia Comaneci-like perfect ten, because that kind of performance would probably cause me to wind up in a cast, or in the hospital. But I have had a couple that I would rate at least an eight.

One of these falls happened when Barbara and I were practicing walking. The doorbell rang. Thinking I was stable on my cane, Barbara rushed to open the front door. As it turned out, I wasn't stable and I crashed down on my back, hitting my head on the sharp edge of a metal table leg. When Barbara returned from the front door, she found me lying in a huge pool of blood—I bled much more because of the blood thinners I'd been taking. I survived the fall, but we resolved to keep our minds on what we're doing in the future, and let doorbell ringers ring away without dropping everything—including me—to answer their summons.

The other major fall I suffered came after my first year of stroke recovery. I had a habit of standing up at the toilet and letting go of the grab bar for a minute in order to pull my pants up. This time I miscalculated, lost my balance, and fell over onto the granite sink counter-top, hitting my rib. It was so painful that I went to the hospital with Deding for an X-ray. Sure enough it was a fractured rib. As I discovered on the Internet, there's nothing you can do when you crack a rib but suffer through it. I took painkillers and rested, and gradually the rib healed.

The most important thing I can say about falls is *don't take chances.* Be extremely careful. In risky situations, like walking over uneven terrain or up stairs, getting in and out of bed, or in and out of cars, try to have someone with you helping you along or providing a steady arm. It's also a good idea for you to wear a gait belt—also called a "transfer belt"(a sturdy two-inch-wide web belt with a metal safety buckle closure) so your helper will have something to hold onto and lift with. If you should fall, a gait belt will be imperative for your helper to get you up off the floor. These belts are available at most medical supply stores. I keep one at home and one in the car.

I really don't like to be helped because I want to be independent, but I do like to have somebody there to hold me up or catch me or pick me up if I make a mistake. You can save yourself a lot of damage—and a lot of trips to the emergency room—if you follow a similar plan.

Osteoporosis Alert

I've been fortunate in that I didn't suffer serious damage in any of my falls. Many people—especially older women—run the risk of fracturing a bone (often a hip) because of osteoporosis. It's an excellent idea for all women of *un certain âge* to have a bone scan. Barbara, who is ten years my junior and has always been *extremely* physically active, was shocked—*shocked*—when during her last physical, her doctor insisted on a bone scan. In the course of the scan, her doctor discovered she was moving into osteoporosis territory.

But all is not lost. Osteoporotic bones can be restored with therapy. Barbara was told to take two calcium-rich antacids twice a day, a 70-milligram Fosamax tablet once a week plus a daily multivitamin that contains vitamin D (a little sunshine wouldn't hurt either).

Safe House

A study by the Injury Prevention and Research Center of the University of North Carolina reports that in one year as many as

20,000 people in this country died in home accidents and seven million were hurt in them. Leading the list of household accidents are falls. Someone who has been disabled by a stroke has an even better chance of becoming a household accident statistic. Some studies have shown that a stroke increases the risk of suffering a fractured hip by up to four times, so we need to do more than the average person to try to prevent them.

Unless you have a friend or family member who is a skilled workperson, making the necessary antifall improvements can be an expensive proposition, and of course your benevolent and protective medical insurance likely won't pay for the improvements. But at least they are usually deductible from your income tax.

First off, if you've lost strength and/or mobility, you should have grab bars installed because you'll need assistance to stand and pull yourself up. My preference is for vertical rather than horizontal bars, because that way you can get a better grasp on them, and no matter how short or tall you are, and no matter if you're sitting or standing, you can reach them. If they're horizontal bars,

---

How to Avoid Taking a Tumble

- If you sometimes feel dizzy when you stand, make sure your dizziness is not a side effect of your medication; if you take more than one, be certain their combined effect doesn't caused vertigo (check with your doctor or pharmacist).
- Have regular vision and hearing tests.
- Wear shoes that give good support and have thin non-slip soles. Avoid wearing slippers and athletic shoes with deep treads.
- Make sure stairwells and hallways are brightly lit.
- In the kitchen, place a rubber mat in front of your sink so you won't slip on spilled water.

they're at one level. I always resent hotels that have just one bar on one side of the toilet because usually it's the wrong side for me. I have to spin around to grab it and then it's not high enough to really pull myself up, so I need help. In your own home you can install them just the way you like. Incidentally, they now make white grab bars, which I prefer to the more institutional-looking metal bars. You should have grab bars everywhere you're likely to go in your house—bathroom, kitchen, bedroom—where you may need help in standing or sitting.

Speaking of bathrooms, one thing that will prove very helpful is an elevated toilet seat. In modern bathrooms the toilets are so low that transferring from a wheelchair to a toilet or from standing to sitting on the toilet can involve a hazardous drop. Fortunately, elevated seats are easily come by in medical supply stores. Rather than those seats you put on and take off, I prefer the kind that you attach semipermanently, because they are more stable. You don't have to be very adept with tools to do this (even Barbara was able to do it!). It's just a matter of a few screws and a glance at the instructions. I have another, portable toilet seat elevator that can be placed over a hotel toilet seat. It's amazing to see the number of hotels that have showers you can roll into with a wheelchair, and bars all over the bathroom, but which have a low and risky toilet seat. You should also have nonskid strips in the bathtub and on the floor of the shower. Don't use bath oils—pleasant though they may be—because they make bathtubs and shower floors slippery.

While not all strokees will need a wheelchair, I am one who does require its services. For those times I need them, I have two wheelchairs. I keep one in the car for transport to places like doctor's offices and to use in hotels, where Barbara pushes it around. I also keep one in the house that I can push around myself because the locks are in the front where I can reach them and not in the rear as they are in the transport chair. It's easy to scoot around at home paddling with my feet.

Now, wheelchairs do not propel very well over carpeting and carpeting can be risky for an unsteady walker. My house was full of carpeting. After my stroke, I had it all pulled up. Fortunately in this old house there were hardwood floors under the carpeting, and that was exactly what I needed. I don't have any loose throw rugs—and neither should you.

The bathroom, on the other hand, was a newer addition and didn't have a hardwood floor, so I had to put in tile, which was expensive. But it looks nice and keeps me able to get around safely on my own, which is my main consideration. I'm continuing to make changes in the house. That's what you should do. Don't delay thinking you'll be back in your pre-stroke shape soon and won't need them. Thinking these kind of changes will turn out to be a waste of money will get you nowhere. If you *do* get better and you *don't* need them, you'll be so happy that you won't begrudge anything you did to make yourself comfortable and mobile and safe in your earlier stroke days.

The Pursuit of Happiness

I've been thinking about happiness. How wrong it is to expect it to last or there to be a time of happiness. It's not that; it's a moment of happiness. Almost every day contains at least one moment of happiness.

—MAY SARTON, *Endgame*

The question of happiness is central to the lives of all human beings—a natural pursuit, a goal we strive for, something intangible that we hope to have more of in our lives than less when the final tally is calculated. But for a strokee—or anyone who has been dealt a bad hand when it comes to health—happiness may often prove more elusive than it might be for others.

Whether you're a naturally negative or positive person, there are ways you can bring more happiness into your life. According to the Declaration of Independence, we have certain inalienable rights. Among these is the pursuit of happiness.

Here are some ways to pursue happiness . . . and to hold on to it. (This is adapted from an e-mail from an optimistic philosopher friend of ours, Cynthia Fena.)

- Happiness is something you decide on ahead of time.
- We have a *choice:* we can spend the day recounting the difficulty we have with the parts of our body that no longer work as they used to, or get out of bed and be thankful for the ones that do.
- Each day is a gift, and as long as my eyes open I can focus on the new day and all the happy memories I've stored away . . . just for this time in my life.
- Age is like a bank account; you withdraw from what you've put in. I can decide every day to deposit a lot of happiness in my bank account of memories.
- I remember every day that to be happy, I can:
    - Free my heart from hatred
    - Free my mind from worries
    - Live simply
    - Give more
    - Expect less
- Whether I like my life or not doesn't depend on how it's arranged— it depends on how I arrange my mind. I can decide to love my life or not. It's a decision I make every morning when I wake up.

A LOOK AT YOUR LIFE VIEW

This simple little quiz will help you see whether you have a positive or negative personal outlook on life, and tell you what that means for your future as a strokee. First take this quiz to discover your natural tendency. Answer yes or no to the following questions.

Quiz 1

Do you watch a lot of TV? _____

Are you known to be a complainer? _____

When you look back on the happy experiences of your past do you now see them as dismal or sad because they are no longer possible? _____

Do you fear medical tests? _____

Do you have feelings of regret over your past life? _____

Do you hate your post-stroke appearance? _____

Are you always moaning about what you cannot do? _____

If you have mostly yesses on quiz 1, your outlook on life is more negative than positive. It's as if you're looking at your life through binoculars, only you're looking through the wrong end. Everything you see is diminished, is much less than it really is. You need to make some attitudinal changes if you are to help yourself to recovery and/or make a successful adaptation to your current situation See Appendix A for books that will be of great benefit for you in changing your outlook.

Quiz 2

Do you have any hobbies or special interests? _____

When you go to have medical tests are you confident that they will turn out in your favor? _____

Do you have a sense of humor? _____

Do you celebrate and are pleased with how you lived your life before-stroke years? _____

Are you generally known to be an optimistic person? _____

Can you still visualize yourself having joyful experiences in the future? _____

Do you have many loving friends? _____

If you have more yesses than nos on quiz 2, you are mostly a positive thinker, in spite of your stroke. Congratulate yourself. You're looking through the correct end of your binoculars, where everything is larger than life.

With that kind of outlook, you have the best chance to heal and thrive. It's very simple. What you hold in your mind is what you'll be likely to experience. This isn't some harebrained scheme of ours: we've been studying it since 1989 when a book titled *Healthy Pleasures* by Robert Ornstein, Ph.D., and David Sobel, M.D., was published. Some quotes that have been helpful to us include:

- "Good health is one result of *joie de vivre*."
- "Good health habits lie not only in your genes, which you can't change, but in your thoughts, which you can."
- "As Abraham Lincoln said, 'A man is as happy as his brain allows him to be.'"
- "The effects of a bright outlook on the future are striking for people facing a major trauma—including . . . a stroke."

You will better contend with your post-stroke problems if you cultivate your garden with flowers of optimism rather than letting it grow over with weeds of despair. Moreover, your new positive attitude will be enjoyable in and of itself for you and—equally important—for all of those around you.

COURTING YOUR LOVE OF LIFE

There are several things you can do to help you enjoy and even love your daily life. Dr. Joyce Brothers spelled out ten of them in an article titled "You Can Lead a More Joyful Life."[7] Here they are, with comments from Barbara.

[7] *Parade* magazine. October 15, 2000.

1. Think that good things will happen. (*This is particularly important for a person who has had a stroke.*)

2. Express gratitude to a loved one. (*Especially if that loved one is your caregiver.*)

3. Put your gripes away in a box. (*Then throw the box out in the trash.*)

4. Be patient with an annoying person. (*Or a person you consider annoying, such as your therapist trying to get you to do your exercises.*)

5. Do something special for yourself. (*It will put you in a good frame of mind so you can do something special for someone else—guess who!*)

6. Reach out to someone who needs comfort. (*Again think of your caregiver, who needs all the comfort he/she can get.*)

7. Focus deeply on each moment. (*And squeeze all the positive feelings out of it!*)

8. Learn from a mistake. (*Acknowledge and appreciate the mistake. It will show you how to avoid it and other mistakes down the line.*)

9. Look closely at a flower or tree you haven't noticed before. (*Beauty is all around you. Focus on it.*)

10. SMILE! It's the best thing there is for all concerned. (*Your caregiver will be particularly appreciative of this and will return your smiles many times over.*)

Make a list of activities or hobbies that you know will make you happy—things that have made you happy in the past, and things you are capable of doing now. Here are a few of my favorite "joy-making" activities.

Cultivate Flowers

I don't mean that literally. You don't have to be out there hoeing and sowing and feeding and weeding. If you can, that's great; but the important thing is to keep flowers in your life, however they get there. Flowers are the quintessence of beauty. They are soothing to have around, and they lift your spirits. That's why people send bouquets to those who are sick or sad. In our home, the rule is to always have a fresh bouquet, or at least a flower or two in a bud vase.

And how is the view of flowers and greenery from your windows? If there is none or very little, try setting out large pots filled with whatever flowers and plants thrive in your state's climate. If there's snow outside your window now, that's okay—it can be a beautiful sight in itself to enjoy until spring comes and brings flowers.

There's a Chinese proverb: "If I keep in my heart a green bough, the singing bird will come." The plants and flowers you carry around inside you are as important as those outside you—perhaps more so. They will comfort you while you wait for that singing bird.

Happy Meals

Eating is a necessity. So why not make it more than that? It's easy to do if you take the right approach and follow the advice of the doyenne of dining, Julia Child: "Above all, have a good time."

If you live in an urban area with all kinds of restaurants, as we do, you're in luck. These days most restaurants offer takeout or delivery, and you can eat very inexpensively that way: no valet parking, less in tips—even when you fling handfuls of change and the occasional dollar bill into the tip jar on the counter. We sometimes get by for $10 for the two of us, often with leftovers!

One thing to watch carefully after a stroke is what kinds of foods you crave. Like subtle personality changes resulting from a stroke, your tastes in food may change slightly. Since a healthy diet is important for strokees—and for that matter, for caregivers who need to keep themselves in good shape—you shouldn't live on fast foods. A craving for fatty convenience meals may rear its ugly head after a stroke. Gil, the father of a young friend of ours, for example, had always eaten fast food in moderation prior to his cerebellum strokes (though one of the first bouquets of flowers in the ICU after his stroke was from the local White Castle, much to his wife's surprise!). However, after his stroke, his fondness for fast food seemed to increase tenfold, and it wasn't long before his pants were getting tight.

That being said, there's no real harm in indulging every once in a while in In-N-Out Burger (the one fast food hamburger the author of *Fast Food Nation,* which chronicles the horrors of fast food production and preparation, will allow his children to eat) or a piece of chicken from Kentucky Fried Chicken (I peel off the skin and crust) or a Subway sandwich or some Chinese takeout from a restaurant that doesn't use MSG. The possibilities are endless and entertaining.

What Barbara and I really prefer, though, is our own home-cooked dishes. Foodies that we are, we often shop at local farmers' markets for the freshest produce, cheese, and baked goods.

But many of us strokees, alas, have problems with chewing and swallowing. If this affects you, it makes it very difficult to dine with others who often prefer beef, pork, lamb, and such harder-chewing meats or foods you can't handle. So what do you do? I stick to what I can chew and swallow, and what's good for me.

Strokee-Friendly Foods

Fruit

Most fruits have soft, fleshy insides that are easy to chew. Other fruits, like apples or pears, can be cut into small pieces. If you still have difficulty, there's no shame in switching to applesauce!

Soups

Any soup is easy if you run it through the blender. For variety, we often eat the soup unblended the first day and blended the following.

Protein

Fish, eggs, turkey, ground meat, or stew meat. One of my favorite proteins is tofu. Another is cheese—especially goat and cottage cheese. Soy milk is also a good source of protein.

Starches

Most breads, except the hard-crusted varieties, are usually no problem. Rice and pasta are enjoyable easy-chewers, as are soft tortillas in cooked dishes or softened in a baggie in the microwave or in a skillet with butter.

Vegetables (Raw)

Tomatoes, avocado, lettuce, mushrooms, cabbage (if made into a finely shredded coleslaw).

Vegetables (Cooked)

Asparagus, cabbage, squash, potatoes (especially mashed), cauliflower, peas, broccoli, spinach, eggplant, tomatoes

Desserts/Sweets

Most people's favorite part of the meal is usually soft and chewable or even melt-in-the-mouthable. A perfect example of this is the Italian delectable tiramisu, which Craig Miyamoto, on his Web site, www.

heavenlytiramisu.com, calls "Heaven in your mouth." Since it's something of a challenge to make, you should seek out a really good Italian restaurant and get one for your strokee's birthday or other special occasion. Other more readily available strokee-friendly desserts include:

- Ice cream and sorbets
- Gelatin desserts
- Custard and flan
- Pudding
- Soft pies (pumpkin, banana cream, etc.)
- Soft cookies
- Cheesecake

One resource that I particularly recommend is *The Easy-to-Swallow Easy-to-Chew Cookbook* by Donna L. Weihofen, R.D., M.S., JoAnne Robbins, Ph.D., and Paula A. Sullivan, M.S. Not only does the book have over 150 tasty and nutritious—and easy-to-prepare!—recipes for people who have difficulty swallowing, it also contains excellent introductory material on swallowing difficulties, which will be important for your caregiver to read.[8]

Music

I spend at least one hour a day—and sometimes two—listening to classical music, which I find extremely calming and comforting. We're lucky, because here in Los Angeles we have two stations that devote themselves exclusively to classical music. So, I never have to hear rock and roll, a kind of music I don't find calming at all. (Two favorite quotes: "Rock is what you call any kind of music you don't like," and "If the music's too loud, you're too old.")

[8]Caregivers should reference "Don't Dis Dysphagia," page 109, of part 2, for information about how to help strokees who suffer eating and/or swallowing difficulties.

I favor the composers of the seventeenth and eighteenth centuries, especially Mozart, Beethoven, and Brahms. I also enjoy early music (Medieval and Renaissance) for the peaceful atmosphere it creates. This music is an important uplifting part of my life.

Music as Therapy

Our appreciation for music comes from the right side of the brain, while our comprehension of language and words is controlled by the left side. Current research is indicating that the aphasia resulting from a stroke on the left side of the brain can be improved by melodic intonation therapy. This kind of therapy can improve speech skills by having patients sing what they want to say—this works, so the theory goes, because people are working from the undamaged side of the brain.

A dramatic demonstration of the left and right brain function is provided by nationally known mezzo-soprano Jan Curtis. She was in the midst of a thriving operatic career when, in 1995, a stroke robbed her of the ability to speak clearly and fluently—in other words, she had aphasia. Her vocalizing, however, was totally unimpaired. Jan could still sing with the best of them, although the songs she sang had to be songs without words. But, putting her career on hold, she slowly, painstakingly learned to correlate the vocal sounds of the lost words with the music that had never left her. Her first return to performing was at the National Aphasia Association's Spring Benefit in March 2001, where she lead off with, "It's a new day, it's a new life for me," and went on to prove it with selections from Gershwin, Porter, and Rodgers. Jan was on her way.

One stop along that way was at the FleetBoston Celebrity Series, where she shared the program with Luciano Pavarotti and Cecilia Bartoli. These two renowned stars received the expected rave reviews from classical music critic Lloyd Schwartz, but he then went on to say, "Yet neither of these got to me as much as the return of mezzo-soprano Jan Curtis, who opened her mouth to sing—gorgeously—five songs (including a devastating 'My Funny Valentine') for the first time on a public stage since aphasia silenced her after the stroke she suffered six years ago."

Laughter

Now we're going to turn to a calming technique that is on a lighter side, one that Barbara and I have always championed and practiced: laughter. We feel it's virtually impossible to feel angry and resentful when you're laughing. Many health professionals agree with us on this. One of the reasons why laughter is such an effective therapy and stress reducer is that when you laugh you briefly relax your muscles—the tense muscles of the body are relaxed, and you have what the British philosopher Herbert Spencer calls a "discharge of nervous excitement." Laughter, according to Norman Cousins, the late editor of *The Saturday Review,* is "a kind of internal jogging" that can be even more health-restoring than really hitting the pavement with your running shoes. Once when Norman was in the hospital with a serious collagen disease, he overheard his doctor say, "I think we're going to lose Norman." This caused Norman to check out of the hospital and into a luxury hotel, where he ate delicious food and spent all day watching tapes of *Candid Camera* episodes. He discovered his laughter from watching these shows helped him have a good night's sleep. The doctors later found, to their surprise, that these laugh sessions had lessened the inflammation in Norman's tissues and—contrary to their dire predictions—set him well on the road to recovery.

You may feel that a stroke is nothing to joke about—and in some cases, this is true. But being able to see the humor in some of the difficult situations you will face can be a balm unlike any other. Laughing just *feels* good. Read funny novels. Check out the

Sunday comics. Listen to *Prairie Home Companion*. Check out a knock-knock book from the library. Or just sit with your family and recount some family memories, some of which are bound to be funny. Do whatever it takes to make yourself laugh, because the cliché is true: Laughter is the best medicine.

Hobbies

I hope you have a hobby, or better still, hobbies, because it's important to maintain vital interests and enthusiasms in your life. People who have no real interests are usually dismal. And the older they get the more dismal they become, because they have nothing that focuses their attention and pulls them up from their dismal depths.

My high school French teacher, who lived to be ninety-six, had an amazing number of interests. In the caregiver section, Barbara will tell you what an avid traveler my teacher was—but traveling was only one of her passions. She was also a lifelong ballet enthusiast, and right up to her last month she continued to attend ballet performances. She also was an avid linguist, belonging to both a French club and a Spanish club in her community of Laguna Beach. Besides that, she belonged to a doll club—she collected international costumed dolls in all her travels. She also grew orchids and had an incredible array of them in her garden. My teacher's lust for life shows how hobbies and interests can help you avoid stress and replace that stress with joy. When you're full of joy, misery and stress simply can't find any lodging!

THE ZEN PATH TO STROKE SUCCESS

I consider myself twice lucky. I'm lucky because I'm still here, despite one major stroke and two minor ones, one major and one minor seizure, and several TIAs. But I'm also lucky because years ago I started studying Buddhism, and it has been of immeasurable help to me in dealing with the aftereffects of a stroke.

So what is this thing called Zen? It's the Japanese form of Buddhism. And what is Buddhism? It is not so much a religion as a philosophy of life, one that is compatible with any religion or lack thereof. Buddhism has at its base a quest for self-knowledge and improved quality of life. The elements of this quiet, calm life philosophy can be of immense help to you as you begin to cope with the realities of post-stroke living.

Attitude Adjustment

In her book *It's Easier Than You Think,* Sylvia Boorstein writes that the lesson of Buddhism is that "it doesn't make sense to upset ourselves about what is beyond our control. The only choice we have is our attitude." It's a tough thing to accept, this lack of control. We spend most of our lives trying to control everything around us, and it's maddening when things occur in our lives that remind us that we aren't in control—like suffering a stroke. Letting go can be scary—but it is also freeing. Your mind is like a bright blue sky, and you can almost feel your body relax once you accept that you can't change circumstance, only your attitude toward that circumstance.

There are four basic Zen practices that promote a right-minded attitude and guide you along the path to happiness, no matter the circumstances you find yourself—including stroke disabilities.

Equanimity

Equanimity is learning to stop all your constant internal churning over this, that, and the other thing, fretting your life away, always controlled by the leaping and chattering and eternal dissatisfactions of your "monkey mind." Equanimity is living with what Zen refers to as "a gazelle's mind," one that is light and agile and graceful. Psychologist Dr. Richard Rubin explains, "Equanimity means balance, the ability to keep yourself together in the face of life's challenges." This is especially important—and difficult—when you are suffering the aftereffects of a stroke and the ongoing fears of having another one. But equanimity also means maintaining inner calm in the face of what the Chinese Taoists call "the one thousand joys and one thousand sorrows of life."

Compassion

Compassion is the art of sympathy in response to suffering. But you must be a Mother Teresa to yourself, too. Show compassion toward yourself when you have difficulty walking or speaking or handling your food. Show compassion to yourself when you have inexplicable outbursts of anger or burst into tears for no apparent reason. Don't blame yourself. You deserve sympathy and understanding, not condemnation. When you treat yourself with compassion, it's easier to have more understanding and compassion for others.

Lovingkindness

There is not anyone in the world who is burdened by too much love. We could all use a little more. As Dr. Rubin points out, "the secret of getting more love is giving more love." The Buddha said that you yourself, as much as anybody in the entire universe, deserve your love and affection. The Bible's "Love thy neighbor as thyself" also means that you should treat yourself with all the love and kindness most of us reserve for others. On a bad day, which many of us stroke people often have, send yourself a bouquet of flowers—and stop to smell them.

Joy

In the movie *Restoration,* a doctor explains to the mental hospital personnel, "You cannot banish Joy, for that is the road to madness." Forthwith, he sponsors a salubrious afternoon of music and dancing for the inmates.

Your first responsibility is to find some time every day to experience joy, no matter what the external circumstances. A Japanese poem says, "The barn has burned; now we can see the moon." Finding reasons for joy during the inevitable barn burns of your life helps you roll with the blows of your stroke situation and not worsen them with stress and anxiety. It is significant that in representations of the Buddha, he is always smiling.

May I here wish you a Buddha smile, a gazelle mind, and one thousand joys to balance the one thousand stroke sorrows you've been experiencing.

GETTING A LITTLE BUDDHISM IN YOUR LIFE

There are many excellent books available on Buddhism. I have two shelves full of them, but I find there are three books I always return to:

- *It's Easier Than You Think: The Buddhist Way to Happiness* by Sylvia Boorstein. Wise and simple teachings that take the mystery out of Buddhist philosophy and help you incorporate Buddhism into your daily life.
- *Zen Mind, Beginner's Mind* by Shunryu Suzuki. Here, along with learning about Zen meditation and practice and how to solve the problems of life, I found my own mantra, which I use to cleanse my mind of distracting and disturbing thoughts. It is *shin ku myo yu*. This is translated as "from an empty mind, a wondrous being."
- *Taming the Monkey Mind* by Thubten Chodron. If most Americans have a chronic condition, it's a monkey mind chattering away in their heads. (Many victims flatter themselves by saying they're "multitasking.") This wise and simple book will calm the

din and give you serenity. Particularly suitable for non-Buddhists who seek understanding of this philosophy.

THE OTHER TEN COMMANDMENTS FOR STROKEES

In closing this part on adjusting to being a strokee and in leading into how to care for a strokee, I will offer you something I stumbled upon on the Internet that may be for you a source of discipline and a reminder to always be compassionate toward those who watch over you.

Ten Commandments for the Strokee

1. Don't ask my caregiver for anything that I can do for myself.
2. Make sure that I thank my caregiver each time she provides assistance to me.
3. Make sure that when my caregiver suggests we go out to eat, shopping, and so forth, I make every effort to go.
4. I will do my best not to complain about my stroke or handicap, or my limitations.
5. I will try my utmost, on my own, to improve my skills, so as to improve the quality of my life and my caregiver's quality of life.
6. Encourage my caregiver to do things on her own, always giving my caregiver some space.
7. I will try to never feel sorry for myself, and I will do my best to keep my sense of humor.
8. I enjoy telling my caregiver that she looks nice, and to me, she is always attractive.
9. I will not live in the past but live for today and the future, learning to live with my new lifestyle, my handicap.
10. I tell my caregiver I love her, because I do.

Jim Kalal, a retired public utility employee in Harlan, Iowa, drew up the preceding "Ten Commandments"[9] after he suffered a debilitating stroke in 1982. These ten commandments have helped him through some tough times coping with being a strokee and have helped him be more graceful when accepting help from his caregiver, his wife.

[9]Originally published by the National Stroke Association, now widely available on the Internet.

A CAREGIVING COMPENDIUM

· ·

CHAPTER 5

Caregiving for a Strokee: The Nuts and Bolts

. . . .

Let me not whine and whimper about things I have no control over.

—HOUSE OF DAVID INTERNET PRAYER OF THE DAY

CONFESSIONS OF A RELUCTANT CAREGIVER

Reluctant caregiver?! Was there ever any other kind? Did anyone, when confronted with a need to give long term-care to a relative or close friend, ever gleefully clap hands and squeal "Oh–Boy-Oh-Boy-Oh-Boy what fun! I get to sacrifice my pleasures and projects and personal life for the twenty-four-seven responsibility for another person?" Not that you'd even consider *not* doing it, especially since the person you're caring for would certainly take on the burden of care-giving if the roles were reversed. In fact if the cared-for one is an aging parent, then they've already given you total care for the years of your infancy and childhood. It's just payback time.

Still, if the truth be told—and it seldom is—every caregiver occasionally turns into a Nurse Ratched, the malevolent, sadistic ogre of *One Flew Over the Cuckoo's Nest,* and every care receiver has moments of being a Sheridan Whiteside, the tyrannical, demanding curmudgeon in *The Man Who Came to Dinner.* The strokee, as June calls herself, has a much less happy situation, especially one who has always been an independent and take-charge person—like June—preferring to give help rather than receive it. If you put yourself in his or her place, you'll see that you have the lesser of two evils—by far!

Still, that's not much of a consolation. As A. E. Housman wrote: "Little is the luck I've had, and oh 'tis comfort small to think that many another lad has had no luck at all." What we have here is a sow's ear that, barring miracles, you're never going to make into a silk purse. All you can do is your best, and some-times you will feel you fall short of even that modest goal.

As It Was in the Beginning

June's stroke struck a couple of weeks after we had returned from a wonderful trip to Amsterdam and Paris. We both agreed it was our best trip ever. June was especially delighted; since she's one quarter Dutch, the Holland leg made her ancestral blood sing.

The night before her stroke, June had had a marvelous birth-day party with friends. The next morning, our computer guru came over in the morning to set up June's computer in the dining room so I wouldn't disturb her while I was working upstairs in the office—and vice-versa. This was the day we were to begin a new edition of our *Diabetic's Total Health Book,* renamed *The Diabetic's Total Health and Happiness Book* since we were going to point out the manifold therapeutic benefits of happiness. The title change was also appropriate because this was a totally happy time for us. We were still infused with the glow of the previous trip and already looking forward to June's birthday trip to Maui. And there's nothing more exciting than starting a new writing project. To paraphrase an anonymous sage, "We had everything to lose because we were happy."

I was working with the guru when June called to me saying that she was "in trouble" and shortly thereafter *it* happened, as described in the introduction.

While June was in her semiconscious state at the hospital, I had nothing to do but worry. This I did with consummate skill and dedication. But as soon as June started coming around, my caregiver duties began.

Initially, these duties mainly had to do with the food at the hospital. After June was taken off the feeding tube, we quickly discovered that none of the hospital food was appropriate for the diabetes diet she had to follow, and certainly not for the low-carbohydrate, high-protein version that she adheres to. In addition, the meals were never served at the right time—especially breakfast (which for June should be between five and six, and for the hospital, was between eight and nine). I won't even comment on the quality and palatability of the food. Anyone who has ever spent time in a hospital can write this dismal scenario themselves! Suffice it to say, I became a one-woman Meals on Wheels, bringing breakfast, lunch, and dinner. In June's case, I looked forward to her return home, where I could more easily prepare appropriate meals. Compared to my delivery service duties, I figured this would be a piece of cake—so to speak.

Of course there were the endless tests—the CAT scans and MRIs—but in June's case, these were not very intrusive and did not cause her much discomfort. This is not true for all strokees. Gil, the father of a young friend of ours who had suffered a stroke, was bombarded almost immediately by nurses and therapists administering cognitive tests while he was still in his hospital bed. There is a very good chance that, as caregiver, your first caregiving duty, aside from vigil-keeping at the beginning, will be to comfort your strokee as he or she begins to realize the magnitude of what has happened to him or her.

Some strokees may slip into denial immediately, believing that he or she did not have a stroke, but rather just ate a piece of bad meat, or overworked him- or herself, and that the effects are temporary. Gil, our friend's father, for example, was convinced that he'd just had a bad reaction to the pistachio nuts he'd eaten for breakfast that day. It wasn't long, of course, before he was convinced that he had, indeed, had a stroke (the CAT scan images of the damaged areas of his brain helped in this). As a caregiver, you should expect emotional responses from the strokee as they grapple with the feelings that are concomitant with any traumatic medical event. Sometimes these feelings can be triggered by some of the cognitive tests that many strokees are asked to take while still in the hospital.

In the case of Gil, being an exceptionally intelligent man, used to being the smartest guy in the room, it was devastating to score less than perfect the first time he took the initial cognitive tests he was given (tests with instructions like "Name as many animals as you can" and SAT-type math questions, for example). Initially, he found fault with the tests, thought the questions were poorly written, etc. Gil couldn't know that, at least for him, the slippage was temporary. While every strokee responds differently, Gil's wife knew to give Gil some "alone time" after these tests, so he could process the fact that the stroke had affected some of his functioning. As a relatively young strokee, too (he was only fifty-six), Gil needed the time to accept the fact that he was mortal, and that no matter how fit and active, no one is immune from the possibility of a stroke. Those first days, though, are a challenge.

Finally, after three weeks, June was told she was going to be sprung. We were both elated, but then something a friend of ours calls "the ka-ching factor" kicked in. Someone in the bean-counting department must have discovered that June could still be covered by her insurance for another week in the hospital, and therefore she was to stay on. I thought June might have another stroke at the news. She had heard from a conspiratorial nurse that "you can always check yourself out." And so—ignoring the scowls and harrumphing directed in her direction by administrative types—she did.

While we began with caregivers on duty for five or six hours a day (more on finding caregivers later in the chapter), I was responsible for June the rest of the time, and all night. Ditto all the shopping and cooking and serving and clean-up after meals, helping June with her insulin injections and blood sugar tests, handling the housekeeping and laundry chores And, as job descriptions always put it, "other duties as assigned."

PREPARING TO CARE

Before you and the strokee leave the hospital, you will likely have a conversation with the rehabilitative physician, or someone from the rehabilitation team, regarding basic care. This conversation depends, of course, on the severity of the stroke your loved one has suffered. Some doctors "interview" family members before releasing the strokee from the hospital, in order to ascertain whether or not relatives can appropriately care for the strokee on the level on which he or she needs care.

If you are deemed able, the rehabilitative physician and nurses should provide you with some basic training. If they do not offer this advice, it is most important that you ask. You will need instruction on the following tasks, appropriate to the kind and severity of the stroke:

- How to help the strokee walk
- How to help the strokee move from his or her wheelchair to the bed, sofa, chair, etc.

- How to help the strokee get dressed
- How to assist the strokee during bathroom visits (baths, visits to the toilet, etc.)
- How to help the strokee eat (managing dining utensils, for example)
- How to help the strokee rest comfortably

Again, if for some reason your doctor or members of the rehabilitation team do not broach the issue or cover it to the degree to which you feel comfortable—if you feel there is still information you need—then *force the issue.*

Resources for Finding Home Health Care

The following organizations will provide guidance for choosing appropriate home health agencies, and, in some cases, provide search engines for finding home health aides in your area. Also check out the Web sites of your state health department for direction.

Medicare Home Health Provider Comparison
www.medicare.gov/HHCompare

National Association for Home Care
www.nahc.org/consumer/wphc.html
(202) 547-7424

Care Pathways
www.carepathways.com/HCx.cfm

Eldercare Locator (U.S. government)
www.eldercare.gov
1-800-677-1116

HELP WITH BASICS

Don't Dis Dysphagia

In the current slang, to "dis" something is to belittle it or treat it with disrespect. A stroke patient's dysphagia—meaning difficulty with swallowing—is something a caregiver should definitely take seriously, especially since it is estimated that 30 percent of all stroke patients and 45 percent of people over the age of seventy-five suffer symptoms of it.

The symptoms to watch for are:

- Trouble with swallowing
- Food sticking in the throat
- Repeated attempts to swallow the same mouthful of food
- Discomfort in the chest after swallowing
- Lack of appetite
- Weight loss
- Frequent coughing during meals
- Grimacing while eating
- Frequently drinking water during meals
- Depositing wads of food inside the cheek (called "pocketing"— June had this problem in her right cheek, the stroke side, in the early days after her initial stroke)
- After-meal tightness in the throat or chest or heartburn or acid reflux

In short, at a time in life or of disability when few pleasures remain, it's a definite diminishment of quality of life to no longer be able to look forward to and enjoy the pleasures of the table.

But it's not simply a matter of losing pleasure; it could result in actually loss of life. Dysphagia has been known to cause aspiration (food and/or liquids entering the air passages). This, in turn, can cause pneumonia. A recent seven-year study of stroke patients revealed that aspiration pneumonia was the cause of death for 20 percent of them during the first year after the stroke and 10 to 15 percent in each subsequent year.[10]

Those statistics should give dysphagia the respect it deserves. What it also deserves is help from a speech and language therapist. While in rehabilitation June was fortunate enough to have the services of two outstanding speech and language therapists. They led her through the three graduated meal levels of the American Dietetic Association's National Dysphagia Diet (NDD), outlined below:

How to Choose Foods and Liquids for Safe, Post-Stroke Eating

Some strokees have no trouble chewing or swallowing; others find it next to impossible. You can adapt this to your strokee's individual needs.

Foods

1. *Pureed.* All foods pureed to a puddinglike consistency with no lumps. We called it "astronaut food" (to take it out of the pablum realm and to give it a little more dignity). Some examples of this would be minced meat with gravy, pureed or mashed vegetables, milk puddings, and soft bread without crust. Lest you be confused, the following, which you might think would fit in this category, do *not:* Jell-O, fruited yogurt, peanut butter, unblenderized cottage cheese, scrambled, fried, or hard-boiled eggs. A *sample menu* could be: pureed chicken, mashed potatoes with gravy, pureed carrots, and applesauce or chocolate pudding. You should do all you can to make this look as close to a normal diet as possible— not an easy assignment.

---

[10] Novartis Consumer Health *Nutrition Matters* newsletter, Summer 2000.

2. *"Mechanically altered" soft foods.* These foods require some chewing ability. In general this category includes foods that are soft-textured. For example: casseroles, fork-mashable fruits and vegetables, bread with crust, ground or minced meats, and some moistened cereals. *Not* included would be items like chewy artisanal bread with hard crusts, dry cake, rice, crackers (and other dry foods), cheese cubes, corn, and peas. A *sample menu* on this level could be: scrambled egg, pancake with syrup, cold cereal flakes with milk, banana, orange juice. (Liquids could be thickened if necessary—see following.)

   Note: Sometimes a mixed diet is prescribed where the patient might have a pureed basic diet but with the addition of one "mechanically altered" food. June, for example, was given scrambled eggs while still on the puree diet.

3. *Normal diets.* This doesn't mean that anything goes. The following should *not* be included: hard fruit and vegetables, corn skins, nuts, seeds, and other hard and crunchy foods. Sticky foods should also be avoided.

Liquids

When it comes to liquids (coffee, tea, juices, and even water), I had thought that the thinner the liquid, the easier it would slip down, and that would be a good thing for a person with dysphagia. Not true. It slips down *too* easily and therefore might go directly into lungland. The National Dysphagia Diet separates liquids into categories: *thin* (thin liquids include water, milk, coffee, tea, soda, ices, and juice or other foods that become liquid at room temperature such as sherbet and ice cream; *nectarlike* (thickened to a nectar consistency such as apricot or peach nectar); *honeylike* (thickened to a honey consistency); and *spoon or pudding thick* (thickened to a pudding consistency). However, the actual viscosity ranges for each category has not yet been determined.

The Dysphagia Diet at Home

It may come to pass that when your strokee comes home, you will need to do some thickening of liquids. Before launching into this project, you should check with the strokee's physician and speech therapist. Once you get an okay from them—along with any suggestions they may have—call Novartis Pharmaceuticals at 1-800-333-3785 and request a copy of their valuable brochure "Guide for Serving Thickened Liquids at Home." If you have Internet access, you can call up Novartis Pharmaceuticals at www.novartisnutrition. com. Once there, click on Contact at the top of the page. Then complete the e-mail form and where it says Questions and Contacts, request a copy of the "Guide for Serving Thickened Liquids at Home." (Actually, this is one case where it's a lot easier and faster just to call for it.)

Several other companies besides Novartis market thickening agents, and the strokee's physician or pharmacist may be able to recommend thickening agents easily obtainable in your area and let you know of any that can be purchased by the case for a discount,

Another possibility, albeit a more expensive one, is to use pre-thickened drinks. These also have the advantage of taking the guesswork and human error out of thickening liquids. Some companies that have these available include:

- *Novartis* (800) 432-3134: Thickened juice, milk, drinks, milk shakes, sugar-free drinks, coffee, and jelled cookies
- *Ross Labs NutraBalance* (800) 986-8502: Thickened water, milk shakes, and juices
- *Hormel Health Labs* (800) 866-7757: Thickened juice, drinks, and milk

Tips from a Pro

Maxine Power, a research training fellow in the Department of Gastrointestinal Science at the University of Manchester Hope Hospital in the United Kingdom specializes in swallowing disorders—in particular dysphagia following a stroke—offers the following tips on achieving optimum nutrition in dysphagia patients:

- Take care when adding thickening agents to liquids. Start slowly and add more, rather than adding too much at once. Some thickening agents such as Novartis's Resource ThickenUp work almost instantly; however, others may carry on thickening for some minutes so that the end consistency may be too thick.
- When adding thickening agents, put the liquid and agent in a capped beaker and shake rather than stir, to avoid lumps.
- As thickened liquids may not always be very thirst-quenching, some patients may not take as many drinks as required to keep them well-hydrated. To help such patients, make a pint of fruity gelatin as this will effectively provide them with a pint of water.

Slow Cooker

Many moons ago when I was first married, slow cookers, especially the Crock-Pot, were all the rage. Everyone rushed out to buy one, believing that this one-pot cooking method made preparation easy and the result delicious. Well, the first part was right, but the deliciousness was questionable, especially since the recipes—usually supplied in a brochure accompanying the slow cooker—mostly all tasted the same. I gradually used my Crock-

Pot less and less until I finally gave it up completely, prefering to go on to more venturesome—and time-consuming—recipes.

But around the time that June had her first stroke there was a slow cooker renaissance. The slow cooker turned out to be a gift of the gods for caregivers and strokees. The caregiver could save long hours in the kitchen and yet enjoy a tasty and satisfying one-dish meal. The strokee could have food that was tender and chewable and comforting, as well as good to eat.

Along with the new name came the publication of a number of Slow Cooker cookbooks that gave the lie to the idea that all things cooked in the slow cooker wound up tasting pretty much the same—a not very interesting same. My favorite big change cookbook is *The Gourmet Slow Cooker: Simple and Sophisticated Meals from Around the World* by Lynn Alley.

Following is a recipe from that book. Like most slow cooker recipes this is as good or better the next day. Since it serves from four to six you can freeze some of it for later use. By the way, the recipes in this are a bit more complex and time demanding than those in the other cookbooks. The author wants you to do such things as grind up spices with a mortar and pestle and brown meats and onions and garlic ahead of time. I don't do the former, and even she admits "that most of the recipes in this book call for an initial sautéing of ingredients to impart some carmelization and flavor. In many cases the outcome of the dish would not be adversely affected if you skipped this step and simply combined all the ingredients in the slow cooker at once."

TARRAGON CHICKEN

SERVES 4 TO 6

*¾ cup plus 2 tablespoons
  all purpose flour
1 teaspoon salt
1 chicken cut into serving
  pieces and skinned
2 tablespoons unsalted butter*

*2 tablespoons olive oil
1 yellow onion finely chopped
1 cup dry white wine
1 cup chicken stock
6 sprigs tarragon
1 cup heavy cream or
  half and half*

- Combine the ¾ cup flour and the salt in a resealable plastic bag. Add the chicken to the bag, several pieces at a time, and shake to coat completely,
- Heat a sauté pan over medium-high heat and add the butter and oil. Add the chicken and cook, turning once, for 8 to 10 minutes, until browned on both sides. Using tongs, transfer to paper towels to drain, then arrange in the slow cooker. Set the sauté pan over medium-high heat and add the onion and the 2 tablespoons flour.
- Sauté, stirring frequently for 10 minutes, or until lightly browned. Gradually add the wine, stirring to scrape up the browned bits from the bottom of the pan. Add the stock and cook, stirring frequently, for 10 to 15 minutes, until the sauce is thick enough to coat the back of a spoon. Pour the sauce over the chicken in the slow cooker and lay the sprigs of tarragon on top.
- Cover and cook on low for 3 to 8 hours, until the chicken is tender. After 3 to 4 hours, the chicken will still be firm and hold its shape. At 6 to 8 hours, the meat will be falling off the bone. Pour in the cream and stir well. Cover and cook for 10 to 15 minutes to heat thoroughly.
- While the chicken finishes cooking, strip the leaves from the

remaining four sprigs of tarragon and chop coarsely. Remove and discard the tarragon sprigs from the slow cooker and stir in the freshly chopped tarragon. Divide the chicken and sauce among plates and serve immediately.

To give you an idea of Lynn Alley's epicurean mind-set, she also recommends a Sauvignon Blanc, Sancerre, or Pouilly-Fuisse as appropriate wines to serve with this dish.

HELPING YOUR STROKEE KEEP UP APPEARANCES

If you've ever watched episodes of the PBS series *Keeping Up Appearances,* you know that most of the humor comes at the expense of Hyacinth Bucket (pronounced, as she says, "bouquet") and her insistence that all the superficial niceties must be observed in every situation. But in reality, keeping up appearances is beneficial for both strokee and caregiver. It builds self-confidence and good spirits, both of which are often in short supply after a stroke. There is scientific corroboration for this. Psychologist Tony Lysons of the University College in Swansea, Wales, studied women in beauty parlors (by attaching electrodes to their heads) and discovered that when a woman has her hair washed, cut, and dried, not only does she look better, but her health is measurably improved. Her morale goes up while her heartbeat slows and her blood pressure goes down by 5 percent.

Hair Dos and Don'ts

It's usually not difficult to find a hairdresser or barber who is accessible by cane, walker, or wheelchair. On the other hand, the strokee may be like June, who prefers to save her energy by having hair taken care of in the privacy of her home. If you don't know someone who makes hair care house calls, ask your friends,

Helpful Hygienic Products

If your strokee finds hair care or oral care difficult to manage on his or her own, you can avail yourself of these products that hospitals use for this purpose:

- *Comfort Rinse-Free Shampoo in a Cap* ($3.49 each) is available in most major drugstores or you can contact Sage Products directly (see below).
- *ReadyBath Shampoo and Conditioning Cap* ($72.59 for box of 30) can be ordered from American Family Medical at (800) 475-8478 or on the Internet at www.amerifamily.com.
- *Toothette Oral Swabs by Sage Products.* These little SpongeBob SquarePants (actually SpongeBob HexagonalPants) sponges on a stick can be used to brush the teeth without the harshness of traditional brushing. They can also be used to swab the inside of the mouth and tongue. Mint flavored. Box of 250 (individually wrapped) $53.68.
- *Sage Perox-A-Mint Flavored Rinse* (8 oz, $12.94). A hydrogen peroxide solution rinse.

You can learn more about the Sage products listed here—and other Sage offerings—by calling (800) 323-2220 or on the Internet at www.sageproducts.com.

or call beauty shops to see if they know someone who does this kind of work. If those approaches fail, you can check with local beauty supply stores for the names of any of their professional customers who will go to a client's house. Incidentally, we find it's usually not more expensive to have hair care in your home; in fact it sometimes costs less, since the circuit-riding beautician doesn't have all the overhead as an in-shop operator.

If the strokee is unable to get into a shower for hair washing, there are a couple of solutions in every sense of the word: Comfort Rinse-Free Shampoo in a Cap and ReadyBath Shampoo and Conditioning Cap. You can use these even when you don't have access to running water. All you need to do is warm the cap in a microwave, carefully following the instructions on the package. You then put the cap on the strokee's head and massage it from the outside for one to two minutes for short hair and two to three for longer hair. This saturates the hair and cleans and conditions it. When the job is done, you simply remove the cap and dry and style the hair. There's no muss or fuss since you throw away the disposable bag (see the product list on page 117).

Since this is written from our perspective, we make it sound as if only woman strokees are concerned about keeping up the appearance of their hair. Not so. It's just as important for men. Everybody likes to look his or her best. Except for those catering to business executives and movie stars, we don't know of any peripatetic barbers, but most women hair stylists do an excellent job of shearing men and most men like having the attention of a woman just fine.

Nails

In our past work with diabetics, who have to be very careful of not damaging their skin and causing infections, we came across Nail Care Plus. This battery-operated device invented in Germany has six tools that file and shape fingernails and toenails. The best part is that it's not possible to cause injury with Nail Care Plus—as you might with scissors or nail-clippers—because the sapphire filing attachments only work on the nails, leaving the skin unscathed. Safe for the strokee and easy for you to use on yourself to keep your own nails in the comfort zone. The Nail Care Plus tool can be ordered from Medicool, Inc. by calling 1-800-433-2469 or visiting www.medicool.com.

Bedsore Loser

Bedsores can develop when there is continuing pressure on the skin, usually from sitting in a wheelchair or lying in bed. The most susceptible areas include the buttocks, the area above the tail bone, heels, back, elbows, and ankles.

The Four Stages of the Bedsore Apocalypse

Whether the strokee is at home or in the hospital or rehab center, it is imperative that you stay on the lookout for the development of bedsores. Bedsores are extremely easy to prevent if you catch them before they start or have reached stage one; they are extremely difficult to cure if they are allowed to progress. If your strokee has any stage of bedsores, be sure to augment the other treatments with excellent nutrition—emphasizing protein—to help the body gain the strength necessary for repairing itself. Vitamin C should also be added and fluid intake should be increased.

Stage One

This is when the skin is unbroken but has reddened areas. These red patches indicate the areas suffering undue pressure, and you should immediately alleviate that pressure by changing the strokee's position in bed (one side, the other side, then the back) every two hours. (More night work and sleep deprivation for you, unless your strokee is capable of turning him- or herself.) You can also use pillows to protect reddened pressure areas such as under the heels, elbows, buttocks, and so on. If the strokee is particularly susceptible to the development of pressure areas, it would be a good idea to get an inflatable mattress (it comes with a pump). Deding got June one of those to use at home, and she takes it with her whenever she has stays in a hospital or rehab center.

A friend of mine who is a nurse in pediatric oncology at the UCLA medical center says that they find medical sheepskin of value to reduce pressure and prevent moisture buildup. She emphasized the necessity of keeping the sheepskin clean. Incidentally, at UCLA they have a skin care specialist nurse who does nothing but prevent and cure damaged skin. When I asked my friend if the majority of this nurse's time is spent working with preventing and carrying for bedsores. Her answer was an emphatic "Definitely."

Stage Two
At this stage the bedsore develops a blister, which may or may not be broken. In either case, you should call your doctor, or, if in a hospital or rehab center, alert the nursing staff.

Stages Three and Four
By these stages, you're encountering serious stuff that you shouldn't handle alone. You need *immediate* help from a health professional experienced in wound care. In stage three, the sore has penetrated all the layers of the skin, making the patient susceptible to dangerous infections. If untreated, stage three rapidly gallops into stage four. In this stage the wound has continued on through muscles and tendons and bone. If this frightens you, it *should,* because the situation becomes life-threatening, especially if the patient is elderly or in a debilitated condition.

The Scent of a Sickroom

It's depressing and distressing for both you and your strokee if the room or even the whole house has the unmistakable odor of sickness. You can always tell a well-managed hospital or rehab facility by the lack of such an unwelcome essence. When June was in the hospital, I noticed that whenever the situation called for freshening the air, they whipped out a bottle of X-O odor neutralizer and sprayed the site. The advantage of this brand over most odor-fighters is that it doesn't try to mask the odor with some sickeningly sweet smell. (Among June's other afflictions, she is allergic to scents of that sort.)

When June moved home I couldn't find X-O odor neutralizer in the stores, so I resorted to my old friend, the Internet: www.xocorp.com; 1-800-442-9696.

This also turned out to be useful when one of the feline caregivers we "employ" had an accident; or, as I prefer to call it, an "on purpose," since they often seem to do it with vindictive intent!

REDUCING YOUR STROKEE'S PAIN

I'm too old to cry and yet it hurts too much to laugh.

—ADLAI STEVENSON (also attributed to Abraham Lincoln)

Strokees may have pain that's either constant or intermittent, or both. June, for example, has pain from the subluxation (partial dislocation) of her stroke-side shoulder, a not uncommon result of a stroke. Aside from being careful when handling the painful or would-be painful area, big-time pain alleviation is the doctor's domain. All you have to do is deliver any appropriate pills if they're prescribed. (Considering the number of pills many strokees take, that's a daunting assignment in itself.)

Equally important is to follow a caregiver's variant of the Hippocratic oath: first cause no pain. Always treat your strokee as gently and carefully as if you were handling a priceless work of art—you are! For example, your fingernails should not be long, sharp talons. Don't emulate Barbra Streisand—see one of her movies if you don't know what I mean. Do emulate Martha Stewart—not her stock market shenanigans, but her nails. I once read in an article that they seldom photograph her hands because the nails are short and show the ravages of her gardening and furniture-refinishing work. A nice middle ground is Katie Couric, short and sensible but still nice-looking. But I warn you, if your strokee is hypersensitive, as many tend to be, you'd almost have to have yourself declawed in order not to occasionally elicit pain with your touch; but in time you'll learn what hurts and will be able to avoid most of it.

Arthur Rosenfeld, author of *The Truth About Chronic Pain*, offers some guidelines for those of us who care for someone in pain. First, he emphasizes that people with pain want to know that you believe in their pain and that you don't think they're just making it up to get attention and sympathy. Along with that he has a number of dos and do nots. Most of these are applicable to other aspects of caregiving, as well as those associated with pain.

- *Do not* judge the person: Pain is not a sign of weakness or bad character.
- *Do* acknowledge the person's suffering.
- *Do not* pretend that you don't notice the struggle.
- *Do* act with respect.
- *Do not* dwell on the future. Pain forces people to live in the present, so make the present pleasant.
- *Do* offer assistance. Ask if there is anything you can do . . . adjust a pillow, make a call.

The rehab center where June spent more than a modicum of time distributed a "Facts About Pain" brochure in which they explained that pain is subjective.

"When a person experiences pain, the pain is as severe and occurs when and where the person says. In other words, logic and common sense do not always apply to pain."

They also suggest some things you can do to help diminish the pain. These include

- Giving the patient a back rub or massage
- Reassuring the patient with comforting rewards and gestures
- Using a gentle touch, which can work wonders
- Playing soothing music
- Helping your patient reflect on pleasant memories

A KINDER, GENTLER CAREGIVER

As a respite from my often acerbic and self-pitying attitude, I think you would benefit from a dose of Laurel's sympathy soothing syrup. Laurel is Laurel Robertson who, with her colleagues at the Nilgiri Press, created an amazing vegetarian cookbook, *Laurel's Kitchen*. They have taken their artistry and experience and fashioned another unique—and necessary—volume: *Laurel's Kitchen Caring; Recipes for Everyday Home Caregiving*. This contains recipes that are a comfort to both the patient and the caregiver, all interwoven with advice on such diverse topics as what to do if you don't eat meat (include a vitamin B_{12} supplement), how to gently coax a reluctant eater, handling the relentless chore of pill-taking, preparing herbal remedies and teas, remaining calm and smiling when your "sickie" (Laurel's term) is irritable, the importance of coming up with little comforts—improvised custom pillows or yet another funny story—and, well, all the information and reassurance and good ideas that you need but didn't know you needed until you read about them. The tone of the book as well as the essence of Laurel herself can be exemplified by this nourishing morsel of her counsel for caregivers:

Hold tight to your sense of humor. Resist courageously when your mind tries to convince you you are wasting your time, not doing a good job, worth more than this, going to have a nervous breakdown, etc., and all the other weasily scenarios our lower self uses to bring us down. Learning to recognize them is an education in itself. Patiently to overcome them, and to keep on helping even when it's hard, is better than college. Afterward, life opens to a different perspective, and very likely you have grown closer to your real self—a happier, kinder, wiser, and more peaceful person than before.

Laurel also realistically faces facts. One dismal fact she told me early on: "You will put on weight. All caregivers do." Right she was. Read on (page 164) to find out the whys and wherefores of my additional ten pounds, what I'm trying to do about it, and what you can do to prevent it.

DISABLING WITH KINDNESS

In Kirk Douglas's book *My Stroke of Luck,* he paints a vivid picture of caregiver kindness gone awry:

> One of the worst things about being the victim of a stroke is that people feel sorry for you. They want to do things for you. And since you also feel very sorry for yourself, you are more than willing to accept their gifts of kindness.
> Your wife says, "Would you like something to drink, honey?"
> "Yes, that would be nice."
> "Don't get up, sweetheart," she says, "Let me get it for you."
> And why not? You've been through a lot. You deserve this loving attention.
> Beware of such temptation. Don't let yourself give in.
> They may not be aware of it, but well-meaning people are encouraging you to become an invalid. They are enablers. Next

thing you know they'll be feeding you and treating you like a simpering idiot. You can't let them.

I found myself fighting a growing dependency on my wife.

"No, honey, I'll get it myself. And while I'm up would you like a drink, too?"

A small thing but it means a lot. When you do that, you feel stronger. You have accomplished something, no matter how small. That's how you cling to your willpower, and you need every ounce of your willpower to get better.

Of course if you've been enabling your head off, it may be a shock to the strokee's system—and to yours—for you to suddenly shut off the customary flow of the milk of human kindness that makes you try to do everything for him or her. No, you'll have to wean off gradually. And as you do you'll often be tempted to backslide when you see the strokee struggle and fumble over a task you could easily jump up and quickly perform. But you must be strong so the one you're caring for can grow stronger. Think Kirk Douglas, grit your teeth, and stay put.

THE STROKEE ROLLER COASTER

According to *The Guinness Book of World Records,* the tallest freefalling roller coaster ride is the Drop Zone at Paramount's Kings Island Theme Park in Ohio. I hate to dispute such a renowned source of information, but the exhilarating highs and plummeting lows at Kings Island are nothing compared to the highs and lows you experience as a caregiver. One day your strokee seems so much better that you're sure he or she has turned a corner on a road to recovery. You're elated, jubilant. You can hardly wait to see what improvements tomorrow brings.

But then tomorrow comes and there are no improvements. In

fact, there is deterioration. From the optimistic highs of the previous day, you plunge into despair. The sad truth of the matter is the higher you go up when things look good, the lower you'll drop down when things look bad.

What you need to aim for is one of the four basic Zen practices—equanimity. (See page 95 in Part 1 for a more in-depth discussion of these practices.) Equanimity means emotional stability, keeping your balance between opposing forces—in this case the highs and lows of the strokee's condition. Equanimity also means maintaining inner calm in the face of what the Chinese Taoists call "the one thousand joys and one thousand sorrows of life."

This is easy for me to say but, I must admit, extremely difficult for me to put into practice. When good things happen I like to squeeze all the "joy juice" out of it and have what I call "an ecstasy attack." But I'm making a valiant effort to walk the equanimity line and put a lid on the highs so I don't bottom out on the lows. Give it a try. It can't hurt and it might help.

TEA FOR TWO

By now you're familiar with the TIA—transient ischemic attack—sometimes, and somewhat incorrectly, called "a mini-stroke." But there is a more common event for stroke victims. June and I call it a TEA—transient emotional attack. I first learned about this from observing my father, who also had a stroke. He, who always had a rather easygoing personality, would sometimes get emotionally overwrought over nothing. I remember when I had been cleaning up my parents' kitchen and came across on old battered paring knife. The blade was dull with rust spots and the wooden handle was bleached out and scratched from years of washing. Since my parents had several other paring knives, all in much better shape, I just threw this relic away. A few days later I found my father rummaging around the kitchen looking for what he called his "favorite knife."

"You don't mean that dull old thing that's been around for years?" I asked. "I threw it away." My father burst into tears. Not realizing that this sort of overreaction is common for stroke victims, I told him not to be ridiculous, this was nothing to get upset about and explained that I'd be happy to get him another knife, a *much better* knife.

"I don't want another knife," he wailed, "I want *that* knife."

Luckily the trash hadn't been picked up that week so I was able to root and rummage around and finally come up with the cherished knife. I learned a valuable lesson, one that held me in good stead when it came to June's "ridiculous" emotional outbursts. (Although I must admit that sometimes I'm caught off-guard and join in a *folie a deux* with June, getting just as overwrought as she in reaction to her TEA outburst.) Try to remember that the emotions are coming not from the person, but from the stroke; and don't take it seriously—or personally. Easier said than done, I know.

I must admit, though, that sometimes I wish June would have had the same kind of emotional change after her stroke that Dr. Howard Rocket did after his stroke, as described in his book, *A Stroke of Luck.* He was *always* optimistic and upbeat—loudly so— and funny. At first his wife had been amused but then she started worrying and wondering: "Was this heightened and sustained optimism and happiness . . . *normal?*"

She asked the doctor about it. He reassured her. "Your husband is on quite a few types of medication, including steroids, which tend to be 'uppers.' Besides which, he has narrowly survived what essentially was the equivalent to a plane crash. It's normal for patients to react emotionally under such circumstances. The technical term for it is 'labile' (changeable). For most people, emotions run the gamut from euphoria to despondence. It's fortunate for all of you that Dr. Rocket seems to exist only at one end of the spectrum."[11]

Yes, it was fortunate, indeed. They had had "a stroke of luck" that I envied.

GIL'S STORY

Strokes are many-faceted affairs. Some are debilitating, as you've seen, but others are not. However, those that do not leave strokees in wheelchairs or using canes still have an effect on the strokee's loved ones. It may be difficult for the caregiver and the strokee's family to get used to the subtle personality changes that often occur after minor strokes. Some of these personality changes have nothing to do with the damaged brain cells: they are the function, instead, of fear. But other slight changes may be due, in fact, to the stroke itself, and the strokee may not realize how these changes affect those around him or her.

Gil, whom we mentioned earlier, is the father of a young friend of ours. He suffered two cerebellar strokes at the age of fifty-six. Up until then Gil had been the very picture of health and vigor— climbing mountains one year, hiking the Alaskan backwoods the next, climbing frozen waterfalls during winters and sheer rock faces during the summers. A veteran journalist, Gil was in better shape than his daughters (though they would never have admitted it) and their weekend pickup basketball games proved as much. But one day, after a "breakfast" of black coffee and a couple handfuls of pistachio nuts, Gil became dizzy and nauseous. He lay down in the bedroom. A few hours later, the room was still spinning, and when he lifted his head even slightly off the pillow,

---

[11]*A Stroke of Luck: Life, Crisis, and Rebirth of a Stroke Survivor* by Howard Rocket with Rachel Sklar.

the nausea was so bad that he began to vomit violently. Soon he could not bear even to open his eyes (these are classic symptoms of a cerebellar stroke).

After a day of near-immobility, Gil finally allowed his wife, Ann, to call his doctor, who suspected vertigo—which, despite its innocuous name, is actually a severe condition that requires immediate medical attention. The doctor told Ann to call an ambulance. One of Gil's adult daughters happened to be home visiting at the time and watched in horror as her vital (and to her, immortal) father was carried out of the house by paramedics on a cot, looking as pale and fragile as a man twice his age.

After some time at the hospital, doctors discovered that Gil had suffered two massive strokes, on either side of his cerebellum. The strokes had been caused by a blood clot that had pushed its way through a hole in his heart, called a PFO (see page 13). There was no physical damage, besides weakness, and Gil seemed lucid. He was placed on Coumadin, and sent home after a few days of bed rest in the hospital. Our friend, Gil's eldest daughter, flew home to "check" on her father, after her mother, Gil's caregiver, had told her that while her father had been spared, there were still some things about Gil that were a little different.

"My father is the most intelligent person I've ever known," our friend said, "and when he is asked to focus on some specific intellectual problem—for instance, a journalism ethics question—it's as if nothing ever happened, and he is as articulate as they come, able to consider problems on many levels of logic and complexity. But then there are these moments when I can tell that things have changed." Gil seemed to his daughter more sentimental, quicker to laugh, and more demonstrative in his affections. He also appeared more impatient, a little quicker to frustrate ("He was always infinitely patient," our friend said), and an avid television viewer (he disdained television programs before). He even speaks much louder now. Ann also finds her husband sometimes to be unusually picky about his surroundings, about the way things are organized in the house. He can be mild and sweet some days, then sharper-tongued the next—typical mood swings in people who haven't suffered a stroke, but unusual for Gil, who was always on a very even keel. The fact, too, that Gil used to be out of the house and at work most hours of every day, and was now haunting their home all day, even if temporarily, was something Ann had to get used to. Ann has found it challenging to know how to deal with her husband post-stroke: because he did not suffer any debilitating physical or brain injury, he is still basically the same person. However, the changes to his personality, though hard for an outsider to see, are very visible for his wife of twenty-five-plus years.

Dealing with a milder stroke is a constant journey—every day will bring different challenges, and every day you will find new, inventive ways to cope. Things often get better, but the new personality quirks will take some getting used to. Our friend and her family have found humor the best tool in dealing with their father's personality changes—and he partakes in the jokes wholeheartedly. They split time into two parts, the way the Bible splits time into B.C. and A.D. When their father does something that once would have been out-of-character, they term it "N.D.": New Dad. The term "O.D." (Old Dad) is used mainly as a reference point ("That's something O.D. would never have done!"). Gil finds this humorous, proving that his stroke didn't change his deeply kind and generous heart.

One other challenge was the way others reacted to Gil. Because he looked so healthy on the outside—no limp, no paralysis, nothing—his friends and fans of his journalism thought he was as good as new. He was asked to accept speaking engagements, something he'd done regularly before the stroke, and to participate in countless charity events. Because he looked so good, people thought Gil was back to his old, mountain-climbing self, and they couldn't understand when Ann gently declined many of these invitations on his behalf. As a caregiver, you may face the same problem. Sometimes the changes a stroke effects can be invisible to friends and outsiders. You, who know the strokee best, may be put in the position of gatekeeper.

Gil had accepted one speaking engagement early on in his recovery and had discovered that big rooms, with their multiple voices and multiple faces, became confusing to him. Everyone develops a kind of brain filter, in which extraneous noise or other stimuli is filtered out so that one can focus on the task at hand (people who suffer from attention deficit disorder have trouble filtering external stimuli); in Gil's case, his strokes had temporarily made large rooms filled with people a little overwhelming to him. He had agreed to give a brief memorized speech before a crowd of 1,700 shortly after his stroke; in the middle of his speech, he recognized a face in the crowd and promptly forgot the rest of his speech.

Gil likens a stroke to having been shot in the head and surviving, having the bullet removed, and then trying to get the brain to heal around the wound. While the neuropathways are healing, they become sluggish, and information is processed more slowly. While Gil improves every day, he has learned not to push it.

MEAN TO YOU

Besides the fleeting transient emotional attacks, there are sometimes permanent, and unpleasant, personality changes as a result of a stroke. Again I use my father as an example. He became mean in both the American sense of the word—nasty, malicious, even cruel—and in the British sense—miserly. This was totally opposed to his normal pre-stroke nature of amiability and generosity.

A friend told me about his brother-in-law, a happy-go-lucky Irishman, the ballad-singing life of every party. After his stroke he was frequently mean to everybody, especially his loving—and much-loved—wife.

While June hasn't had a huge personality change, she does have her moments of unkindness in which she makes mean and hurtful remarks. Luckily—I guess!—these are usually only directed at me and not to other friends or associates who are unaware of any changes of this sort. And as for meanness in the British sense of the word, that is nowhere in her post-stroke psychological makeup. On the contrary, she spends a lot of time thinking of ways she can donate things and money to people and organizations in need. From remarks she has made, I think this has something to do with her stroke-engendered feelings of mortality. She wants to do these not-so-random acts of kindness while she's still here to do them. This is something we would all be better off emulating with or without the goad of mortality feelings.

The one thing a caregiver has to beware of is reacting in kind to the meanness of the strokee. That only makes matters worse on both sides. Just quietly count to ten or twenty or whatever it takes and figure this, too, shall pass if you don't exacerbate the situation.

COMPLAINT DEPARTMENT

There's one thing you'll learn to never, *ever* do: complain. At least in front of your strokee. You can't complain to strokees, because feeling the complaint is being directed toward them, which in a sense it is, they will react in one of many counterproductive ways.

They may cry, become enraged, threaten suicide, or give you a prolonged silent treatment. They can also play the game of "can you top this complaint?" This is a game you'll always lose because, feel put upon and whimper as we may, we all have to admit that the strokee has it much worse and has much more to complain about.

You can't complain too much to friends or you soon won't have any left to complain to. You can't complain to doctors and nurses and other health-care people. They're always too overworked and harried to listen to whining and grousing caregivers. As it is they hardly have time to attend to the business at hand.

Most of all you can't complain to yourself. Although you are a sympathetic and willing listener and agree totally with your litany of complaints, if you dwell on the hardships of your life you pull yourself ever downward into the depths of despair. Often, you're the only person you can rely on to cheer yourself up. And you certainly can't cheer up your strokee if you're always inwardly chewing the complaint cud.

That being said, however, keeping everything bottled up inside is not a good tactic either. This is where support groups come in handy. There is likely a support group in your community that you may find helpful and healing; knowing that you are not the only person going through this kind of difficulty can be a million-dollar balm (see page 142 for support group resources).

COMPLAINTS WITHOUT WORDS

You can deliver complaints without saying a word, and they can be as hurtful and discouraging as the most eloquent of verbal lamentations.

Sighs

When I was just out of college and working at my first library job, I had a bad case of Weltschmerz and *mal du siecle,* those post-adolescent pangs you're subject to when not liking where you are and unsure of the future. My major symptom of this condition was constantly "sighing like a furnace." It became a joke around the place. One of the library clerks started calling me "Cap," the name of her black Lab who had the habit of heavily sighing as if his dog life were too much to bear.

With Cap's help I got over sighing for many years, but the bad habit returned to me full force in my role as caregiver. When I realized what I was doing and the effect it had of creating an atmosphere of gloom, I called on Cap for assistance to get me over it. When a sigh started to escape my lips, I would say to myself, "Cut it out, Cap." It usually worked. I offer it to you as a sigh-eradicator.

Put on a Happy Face

Even worse than sighs are dismal facial expressions. While sighs may come and go, your gloomy face is always hanging out there, telling the world and, more to the point, the strokee how miserably unhappy you are. What can you do about it? You can't wear a mask or put a paper bag over your head. What you *can* do is pretend to be happy. Follow the message of Kurt Vonnegut's novel *Mother Night:* "Be careful what you pretend to be, because in the end, you are what you pretend to be." Keep a smile on your face, or at least a pleasant expression. After a while you may find, to your surprise, that it lifts your spirits—not to mention those of your strokee. Or, as a shortcut, tell yourself a joke right before you walk into the strokee's room. Better yet: Share the joke!

Making Decisions

There was the story of the grapefruit sorter who had a nervous breakdown. It wasn't that the work was so hard. It was all those decisions. Many strokees are like the grapefruit sorter. They have difficulty making decisions, even the simplest ones ("How would you like your eggs fixed? "Do you want to take a nap?" "What TV program would you like to see?"). This makes it very hard on the caregiver. If you don't ask and instead make the decision yourself, you may be greeted by a "No, no, no" (on the verge of tears), "*that's* not what I want." If, on the other hand, you pass on the decision-making to the strokee, you are often met with silence. After waiting a while, believing that your question hasn't been heard, you raise your voice and ask it again. This irritates the strokee in the extreme: "I'm *thinking.* You don't need to shout. Just give me some time."

As with so many caregiving situations, it seems that whatever you do turns out to be the wrong thing. I wish there were a simple solution to this problem, but if there is I haven't found it. It's a matter of staying relaxed, not getting upset, and letting the decisions—wrong or right—fall where they may.

Dinner Time

I once read an article that said that to a dog, dinner is the high point of the day. If you have ever had a dog I probably don't have to tell you that. Your dog may be limply lying there looking morose, but when he hears the old familiar sounds of his dinner preparation, he perks right up and dances with joy and excitement and anticipation. I venture to guess that dinner may be the high point for a lot of us humans, too—a hot meal at the end of a tough day, the welcome company of a family or friend, that nice, full feeling afterward.

Strokees are no different—but sometimes they know how to double or triple (or even quadruple!) the pleasure by asking for meals several times a day, often at totally inappropriate times.

When June sounds the alarm, as a conscientious caregiver I usually manage to rustle up something to assuage her so-called hunger. The reason I refer to June's "so-called hunger" is that it most likely isn't real hunger that needs assuaging, but something else. It could be loneliness, and having someone serve you something to eat gives you the company and attention that you crave. It could be sadness, that post-stroke empty feeling inside that you long to fill. But my money is on boredom. The challenge is finding something that he or she wants to do that doesn't involve food and that is feasible. June, for example, would probably not keep longing for food at all hours if she could go to a play or a concert or hop on a plane for San Francisco or Paris. But since at this time she can't, I have to keep dredging up possibilities, such as calling a friend, encouraging her to go through the book review section of the *Los Angeles Times* or *New York Times* to select books she'd like to read, bringing in a video or DVD that I think she'd enjoy (I usually strike out on that one as she's very hard to please on movies), having her sort through the myriad catalogs that arrive in the daily mail and see if there's something she'd like to order. If one possibility doesn't work, I keep trying, and so should you. If a possibility works one day and then doesn't work the next, don't give up, try, try again. Unless you want to become an around-the-clock short-order cook on top of all your other duties and chores, you must find other ways than food to keep your strokee entertained and interested in life and the many pleasures it contains despite the limitations that a stroke may have imposed.

As an aside, June's sense of humor is alive and well, and she's quite aware that she has a food fixation. When she approaches the table she often announces: "Here comes the eating machine."

And the strangest part is that despite her marathon eating, June hasn't gained an ounce. As her doctor says, "That's a problem we'd all like to have. Let her eat all she wants."

HELPING BRAIN CELLS RECOVER

The Strange Case of the Baby in the Lumberyard

I've heard from various therapists that it's important to keep the strokee's brain cells perking (perk: to become lively, cheerful, or vigorous) and restoring themselves.

They suggested such things as keeping bright colors around (even in your own attire), playing music, turning on simulating programs on the usually much maligned television, and most important engaging him or her in conversation or playing word games.

I particularly like this last one, and I came up with a question-and-answer game in which June had to respond appropriately to such common cliché phrases as:

Hard as?	June: nails
Happy as?	June: a lark
Clean as?	June: a whistle
Frisky as?	June: a colt
Drunk as?	June: a skunk
Busy as?	June: a bee

If June couldn't come up with an answer I'd tell her, and then later—usually the next day—I'd ask her again and she almost always got it right.

In time I started to throw in some embellishments like,

How did you sleep last night?	June: Like a baby.
How are you going to sleep tonight?	June: Like a baby.

Then I got tricky with pointing out that there is another answer to "How are you going to sleep tonight?" or "How did you sleep last night?" It's "like a log." She acknowledged the truth of that and for a while alternated between the two answers. This inspired me to get *really* tricky:

How are you going to sleep tonight?   June : Like a baby.
And where is the baby?

That stumped her, so I informed her that the baby was on a log; it's a double-whammy ("sleep like a baby on a log") description of a good night's sleep.

June used that response for a while and then one morning this exchange took place:

How did you sleep last night?   June: Like a baby.
And where was that baby?   June: In a lumberyard.

In a lumberyard?! How did she come up with that? Then I finally figured out that it showed how a recovering brain works. A log is wood. Wood is made into lumber. Lumber is kept in a lumberyard. *Voila!* It makes perfect sense. It also injected some humor into our game.

Now it's always "How are you going to sleep tonight?" to which June replies: "Like a baby in a lumberyard." Then one day when I was rippling through the standard questions and answers, I asked the familiar "fat as " expecting, of course, "a pig." Not so. June smiled evilly and answered: "An American." With that I realized that she was on her way to becoming her old self.

These games can be very idiosyncratic, very personal to you and your strokee. They needn't make a whole lot of sense to anyone else, so long as you, as the caregiver, can tell that the strokee is using his or her brain and re-training those neurons, re-treading the neuropathways.

CHAPTER 6

Taking Care of the Caregiver

. . . .

The physical and emotional wear and tear must have started to show. Friends, after inquiring about June's well-being, would look at me searchingly and say, "How are *you* getting along?" They looked dubious at my, "Oh, fine." One of them, my no-nonsense businesswoman friend Noeleta, wouldn't accept that answer.

"Look," she said, "You have to take care of yourself. If you break down, the whole house of cards collapses." When she put it that way I realized—and I hope you will too—that your first and foremost duty has to be to keep yourself functioning physically and emotionally. Although the strokee is the major focus of your attention, when you are number two, as tradition has it, you must try harder. Part of that trying has to involve keeping yourself healthy and happy. This may turn out to be your hardest job of all.

One of the most important things to do is to reach out to others. With stroke the leading cause of disability in the United States, and growing even more common as the Baby Boomers age, there are likewise more and more caregivers coping with taking care of their strokee. Having an outlet for your fears and frustrations can be invaluable.

SUPPORT GROUPS FOR CAREGIVERS AND THEIR STROKEES

Back when we were laboring in the vineyard of diabetes we were often invited to speak to diabetes associations. In our talks, we always wholeheartedly recommended diabetes support groups. At the end of one of our presentations a woman sidled up and said, "Frankly, I don't think much of those support groups."

"Why is that?" I asked her.

"Well, it seems to me that it's just a bunch of people sitting around complaining."

She just didn't get it. One of the main virtues of a support group is that it gives you a chance to vent your spleen and clean out your woe-clogged pipes with impunity. No one who isn't going through the same things you are would sit through such a gross and—to them—boring display of embarrassing emotions. You'd have them racing for the door. But in a support group you'd have their rapt attention, and at the end probably be rewarded with a round of empathetic applause.

But that being said, airing complaints is not the true purpose of support groups. They exist mainly to help strokees and their caregivers and concerned family members and friends learn more about strokes, forestall future strokes, share their experiences, and encourage and inspire each other to continue to work toward more recovery and a better quality of life after stroke. It can even be a place to make friends and socialize with them at a time in your life when a friend is very much in need and hard to find, as this Dear Abby correspondence shows.

Last February my husband suffered an anoxic brain injury (lack of oxygen to the brain). Needless to say, he is no longer the man he was.

Our friends have all disappeared. They tell me it's hard for them to see him like this. How do they think I feel?

Am I wrong to feel hurt? I don't know why they can't even call. Talking has always been an outlet for me, but no one ever calls me anymore.

No one knows how someone else feels until they've been there, but what happened to, "I'll be there for you" or "Call me if you need me"?

Is it normal for people to avoid friends when they are in trouble or pain?

Friendless in Georgia

Dear Abby's response was her usual combination of sympathy and practicality. She said that what Friendless's friends were doing was "human," "common," and "cowardly." But in effect, she advised her to, as New Yorkers put it, *fuggedaboutit*. She pointed out that rather than dwelling on how her supposed "friends" had let her down, her time would be much better spent with a support group with whom she would have much more in common.

COPING WITH DEPRESSION

. . . that cruelest of torments inflicted upon the sinners of Dante's Inferno; the remembrance of past happiness recalled in present sorrow.

—BENITA EISLER, *Chopin's Funeral*

In Sue Shellenbarger's *Work and Family* column in the *Wall Street Journal,* she tells of a woman who is the caregiver for her elderly stepfather with Alzheimer's.

Finding Support

A number of organizations offer support and information for overwhelmed caregivers, including where to find a stroke caregiver support group in your area (some sites even provide instructions on how
to create a support group!).

- American Stroke Association's "Warmline" (Stroke Family Support
  Network). The folks who answer the phone here are often caregivers themselves:
  1-888-4-STROKE (1-888-478-7653)

- American Stroke Association's Support Group Finder (simply type
  in your zip code and a list of the stroke support groups in your
  area will pop up!): www.strokeassociation.org/strokegroup/

- The Caregivers' Support Group: Don't underestimate the power of
  the Internet when it comes to finding emotional support. MSN's
  virtual caregiver's community was originally started for those taking care of transplant survivors, but it has grown to include caregivers cut from all cloths. The site provides advice, a bulletin
  board, tips, and so on.
  www.groups.msn.com/TheCaregiversSupportGroup/

- Caregiver-Information: another wonderful Web site, which provides information for caregivers, along with a way to connect with
  other caregivers.
  www.caregiver-information.com/

- Generation S: a site for young victims of stroke (an underreported
  phenomenon) and those who take care of them. Provides lots of
  great information, along with a bulletin board where you can meet
  an "e-buddy" who can support you through the tough times.
  www.orgsites.com/pa/generation-s/index.html

- Faith in Action: Faith in Action is an interfaith volunteer caregiving
  program that provides grants to local groups representing many

faiths who work together to care for their neighbors who have long-term health needs. Faith in Action volunteers come from churches, synagogues, mosques, and other houses of worship, as well as the community at large. Volunteers help those in need by providing non-medical assistance with tasks such as picking up a few groceries or running errands, providing a ride to the doctor, friendly visiting (talking and listening), reading, or helping to pay bills.

Phone: (877) 324-8411

www.faithinaction.org

- CareSsentials: Exclusively for caregivers, this Web site is maintained by an apparently indefatigable woman named Jo Cavanaugh. She leads off her site with, "Do you wish that your life was different?" (A rhetorical question if ever I heard one!) She lists all that she has available to help caregivers find the "peace and fulfillment" that she has plus the information we all need. You should definitely sign up for the "Caregiver Tips" e-mail newsletter. But for what we're here concerned with—support groups— she has one we can all attend no matter how already overburdened our schedules are: a telephone support group called Caregiver Connection. It meets once a week on Wednesdays at 10:00 P.M. EST. As she says, "Sign up now [on her Web site]. Take time to recharge. Make time for you."

www.careSsentials.com

"Her setup isn't a happy one," Shellenbarger writes.[12] "She rarely gets out of the house. Her voice breaks as she talks of the past, when she could jump in her car anytime to visit her adult children."

---

[12] *The Wall Street Journal,* June 21, 2002.

As I think of the freewheeling past days of travel, I know exactly how she feels. I remember how we were all set to go to Maui when June's stroke hit. I pretty much took that in stride because I was sure that with enough physical and occupational therapy, we'd be on the road again. After all, we hadn't let diabetes or a shattered tibial plateau stop us. In fact we—or at least I—had it all figured out that we would celebrate June's recovery by going back to Paris and walking the length of the Champs Élysées just as we had done on our last trip. And it all seemed to be happening. June could walk from the hospital parking lot to the therapy center and then do some more walking there. She had a wheelchair, but only used it intermittently. We took a couple of trips to Santa Barbara and she was able to walk to and from the hotel dining room and take a turn around the garden. We stayed overnight in a couple of local hotels for the travel practice, and I remember two days before her second stroke she walked from the parking structure to the doctor's office with only a cane and a lean on me. The doctor's wife/receptionist was amazed and delighted with the progress June had made. But then the second stroke did its nefarious thing.

After that it was back to therapy square one, and June was not progressing as before. When we tried to go back to Santa Barbara, June found she wasn't up to walking with her cane, and although she had a wheelchair with her, it was difficult to negotiate on the carpet. It was even more difficult to get out of bed without the electronic bed she had at home. No walking took place in the restaurant or the garden. She missed the help of the grab bars she had installed at home after her first stroke. We checked out a day early.

It was obvious that June was now only comfortable and confident and happy at home. She had also lost her former enthusiasm for therapy. She had a "been there, done that and what good did it do me?" attitude and, against my protests, dismissed all her visiting physical and occupational therapists, figuring that she and her then other caregiver, Deding, could do as well—or as poorly—on their own. It gradually dawned on me that the Paris walk might never take place, and neither would any of the many other trips we had planned.

With this realization I became very depressed and couldn't even read travel sections of the *Los Angeles* and *New York Times* or listen to "The Savvy Traveler"—a program I previously never missed—because they made, as the Calypso song puts it, "watuh come to de eye." So did postcards from traveling friends. So did ecstatic messages from our longtime friends who had moved to the Napa Valley and whose lives were now a glorious cycle of wine-tasting and picnicking, and sightseeing and impromptu excursions to San Francisco or Mendocino or to Biba's in Sacramento for lunch or to wherever their whims took them. Their every communiqué ended with, "It just gets better and better." All this when as far as I was concerned it just kept getting worse and worse.

Schadenfreude is a German term meaning "delight at the misfortune of others." I was experiencing the opposite "unhappiness caused by the joy of others." I wondered if there was a German word for that ignoble emotion so I called up the *Ask Jeeves* search engine on the Internet and, lo, I was not alone. Other people had asked the same question. It turns out there is no such term, but someone offered up an original: Freudenschade and I adopted it as my personal watchword.

June took to screening all happy letters and e-mail messages and postcards with ecstatic messages lest they make me sink into a funk. But that didn't help. Just about anything could bring me down, even looking in a kitchen drawer and seeing the Farmers Café and Lounge shot glass, which brought back memories of one of many ski trips. The glass was given to us by the owners of the place when they gave us a ride into Steamboat Springs after I almost skidded the car off a steep cliff on Rabbit Ears Pass, only to be miraculously stopped by a snowbank. Ah, those were the days!

Our wonderful travel agent, Maggie, kept inviting us to San Francisco to see her new—actually now year-old—baby. She had even arranged for an amazing bargain rate for us at one of San Francisco's best hotels. She was also still holding onto our paid-for Maui hotel and plane reservations.

The ironic part was that the friend who died just before June's stroke had left her a sum of money, which she stipulated should be used for travel. She was a great traveler herself, having been to China three times and around the world on a freighter, and to Europe and Asia and South America too many times to count. The woman had even seen such now impossible-to-duplicate destinations as pre-war Berlin. She and her architect husband had restored a house in Antigua, Guatemala, and they spent several months there every year. She had had it all, and yet it wasn't enough. In her early nineties she kept planning trips that fell through at the last minute because of health problems.

"Jeez, what does she want?" I thought. "She's been everywhere in the world twice over." Well, she, like Oliver Twist, wanted more. Now I totally understood her feeling.

I've had way more than my fair share of travel and I shouldn't complain. But still, I couldn't keep these feelings of sadness and loss and longing away when I thought of the wonderful trips of the past. I tried to analyze it and discovered that these feelings were identical to the way I felt when I went away to summer camp for the first time. I was carrying around a great internal sorrow that I couldn't get rid of. I thought of this collection of emotions as "The Summer Camp Syndrome." Even if you've never been to summer camp you've probably experienced these feelings at some time in your life and you may be experiencing them again here and now and with greater intensity in your caregiver role.

For me, it was the loss of my freedom to travel. For you, it may be something else: lack of time to garden, for example, or a pottery class you had to drop. Your life has changed, too, and these changes may be difficult for you to deal with, at least at the beginning. Allow yourself to mourn. But, if time passes, and you find you are not improving, take it as a warning sign that perhaps steps need to be taken to remedy the situation.

In my case, my depression was a virus and June was catching it. She started saying that she had ruined my life by taking away the one thing I most desired. She, who, after the stroke, had always been upbeat and full of happy-just-to-be-alive feelings, grew almost as morose as I. Maybe it was time for professional intervention.

SHRINKING SORROW

I've always thought I should have a lot more money than I do because I don't smoke and have never been to a psychotherapist, both very expensive activities. The only reason I thought about it now was that I had been talking on the phone to a woman in Pennsylvania whose husband had had a stroke. Strangely enough, his stroke struck the night before they were going on a trip to Greece. The woman felt it was a miracle that it happened when they were still home and he could get prompt medical attention; otherwise, he might not be alive today.

When we were comparing notes on our caregiver roles, I was embarrassed to confess to her that my biggest problem was being very depressed over the fact that I couldn't travel. She didn't seem to think that was ridiculous at all. Along with her losses of time for seeing friends and going out to movies and the theater, attending her club meetings, she, too, missed all the travel she and her husband had done in pre-stroke days. Then she asked, "Have you

Coping with
Caregiving-Induced Depression[13]

- Depression is fighting reality. Reality will defeat you every time. As long as you fight reality you will be depressed. Acceptance now! All depressions eventually end because you ultimately have to give up.

- Give up the fight. Although a surrendering nation thinks the future will be terrible, nations often do better after the surrender. Look at Germany and Japan after WWII.

- Take the energy that you're wasting fighting reality and work with reality rather than fighting against it. You won't lose hope, you'll actually have more hope. Hope for something that is possible rather than impossible.

- Keep expectation low, motivation high. Have limited expectations but infinite hope. Stay optimistic. (People are naturally optimistic.) Eliminate the negative. When you're negative you're telling yourself some kind of lie about the future. Question those thoughts.

- A caretaker always has a degree of anger. Expect ingratitude. The more you do, the more ingratitude you get. People don't like to be dependent. They want an equitable relationship. Think of the prodigal son.[14]

- You can't be paid twice. The pay is in doing the deed. You can't expect to also be paid with appreciation, gratitude.

- Humor is where pain meets truth. Humor helps you accept the truth of the pain.

- Happiness is love. Love the angst you feel. It's part of you. It's part of life. Love the stroke person's paralyzed arm in its strange position. Every part needs to be loved. To understand anything, love it.

[13] From Dr. Gary Emery.

[14] Dr. Emery admits to being a kind of prodigal son. His brother stays home and cares for their aging parents. When he comes home on one of his infrequent visits, he's loved and treated like a prince. Mother bakes pies. Brother says, "Why don't you bake pies for me?"

tried going to therapy?" Well, no I hadn't. She said she thought it would do me a lot of good.

I was dubious. I had neither the time nor the inclination to lie around on a couch discussing my toilet training. But it did set me to thinking. Maybe, just maybe, some therapy would help. I had heard of cognitive therapy. Someone once described it to me by giving me the example of, say, a person had who a fear of crossing the street. The therapist wouldn't try to analyze the reason why she had this problem by probing—possibly for years—all the events in her life since infancy. No, the cognitive therapist working with her would—and usually very quickly—make it possible for her to cross streets without fear.

To find the appropriate therapist for me, I turned to a friend who for years had regularly gone to a psychotherapist of the lie-on-the-couch style. But when she had a problem for which she wanted immediate action, something like the fearlessly crossing the street example described above, she turned to another therapist—a cognitive therapist. I got his name and phone number and made an appointment.

Cognitive Therapy Notes

I had a total of four sessions with Dr. Gary Emery. When I came home from these appointments, I made notes of what I remembered from the sessions (something I suggest you do as well—the notes will be helpful for you to refer back to during difficult spots).

For me, the sessions with Dr. Emery helped ease my feelings of sadness and loss; this is not to say that I was suddenly skipping around with a smile on my face and a song in my heart, but neither was I the melancholy baby wearing a mask of tragedy that I was before. I even started reading the travel sections and listening to "The Savvy Traveler" again. No longer was I engulfed in waves of "Freudenschade" at reports of my friends' joyful experiences.

Well, maybe I still felt a twinge now and then, but usually I could quash it and get on with my life.

Along with a headful of more positive thoughts, Dr. Emery gave me some business cards with a difference: On one side of the card was one of his mottos, such as the ever-appropriate "Expect ingratitude." On the other was a list of four questions to ask yourself whenever a depressing or discouraging thought enters your mind:

1. Can you really know that it is true?
2. Is there any good feeling or reason to keep this thought?
3. Who would you be without this thought?
4. Can you turn this thought around?

For a more coherent and specific version of Dr. Emery's thoughts and methods of treating depression, and a list of his publications and tapes, you can check his Web site: www.rapidcognitivetherapy. com. If you prefer to seek out a living, breathing, hands-on cognitive therapist, you can request information on cognitive therapists in your area from the University of Pennsylvania Center for Cognitive Therapy: www.uphs.upenn.edu/psycct or phone: (215) 898-4100.

THE TWO ROADS TO CURING DEPRESSION

There are two ways—generally believed to be equally effective— to treat depression: cognitive therapy, which we've just discussed, and medication.

Cognitive therapy is considered a top-down approach because it focuses on the cortical, or top part, of the brain, the area associated with thinking, recognizing, and changing despondent moods and negative thoughts. On the other hand, antidepressants work from the bottom up, concentrating on the limbic area around the hypothalamus that is involved with emotion and memory.

A Deeper Shade of Blue

It is estimated that in this country, nineteen million adults are plagued by clinical depression. Are you one of them? Probably you—as I did—feel that your depression is as about as bad as a depression can be. But Dr. Gail Saltz, assistant professor of psychiatry at the New York Presbyterian Hospital Weill-Cornell School of Medicine, reporting on the *Today Show* offered ten signs to help you figure out if you are just sad or are truly depressed:

"If you have half or more of the following symptoms for more than two weeks, or if any symptoms are impairing your ability to function, then you may have clinical depression.

1. Persistently sad, anxious, or empty mood.
2. Sleeping too little (awakening in the early morning and unable to go back to sleep) or sleeping too much.
3. Lost appetite or increased appetite.
4. Not able to enjoy any activities, lack of interest in doing anything.
5. Feeling restless or irritable.
6. Difficulty concentrating or being decisive.
7. Feeling exhausted.
8. Feeling hopeless, helpless, and worthless.
9. Physical problems that have no medical cause like headaches or stomach aches.
10. Thoughts of death or suicide.

Depression may look different in different people. One may be slow, exhausted, feel numb and utterly hopeless while another may appear anxious and irritable. These are both signs of depression but different kinds and a professional will need to determine which it is in order to recommend the proper treatment.

Which Road Do You Take?

If you or your therapist ascertain that you aren't suffering from clinical depression, you may instead be embroiled in your own version of my "summer camp syndrome," a condition in which you'll be able to at least take the edge off your feelings of sadness and loss by reading books and listening to tapes on cognitive therapy. And don't forget two other old stand-by palliatives—exercise and a sense of humor. Even just talking with sympathetic friends or relatives about your situation can sometimes help. They may be able to offer some ideas on how to make things better for you.

But if your depression deepens and you begin to feel incapacitated by it, it may be some comfort to know that there are other possibilities you can explore, including a combination of cognitive therapy and antidepressants.

The Time Cure

Another comfort—albeit a cold one—is that over time you will probably feel better than you do at this moment. The first year is the hardest. After that, little by little, it gets progressively less arduous. This is not to say that you ever move into a zone of perfect comfort and contentment with your life as a caregiver; but you eventually learn enough tricks of the trade to make it easier to handle physically and emotionally.

SECRETS OF A LONG LIFE

When you're feeling blue, honey, do something nice for someone else.
—T. JEFFERSON PARKER, *Red Light*

The Institute for Social Research at the University of Michigan studied 423 men over the age of sixty-five and their wives. This study revealed that those who provided physical and/or emotional help to a spouse or a person in another household were only about half as likely to die in the five-year period following the study as those who did not provide such support.

Dr. Stephanie Brown, the psychologist who led the study, explained that this substantiated previous research on the positive effects of social contact on mortality. Strangely enough, Dr. Brown emphasized that "What is beneficial about being in a close relationship is rooted in the contribution we make, not in the support we receive from these individuals." In other words the findings emphasized the importance of being needed, of feeling useful. And, we caregivers definitely feel needed and useful because, of course, we are!

Short-Term Benefit

There was this woman, who, despite her advanced years, had a lovely, flawless complexion. What was the secret of her dermal success? She had agoraphobia (from the Greek for "fear of the marketplace"). People with this psychological condition have an abnormal fear of being in crowds, public places, and open spaces. Hence, they stay at home indoors all the time. If you want to see how nice your skin would have looked with the benefit of agoraphobia, take a look at your bare stomach.

Caregivers have a kind of involuntary agoraphobia in the sense that they're pretty much confined to close quarters. Since June's first stroke I have never had a cold, nor have I had a bout with the flu, despite the fact that there have been some minor epidemics going around. Neither have I felt I need to worry about other communicable diseases. This is because I'm seldom if ever out in crowded theaters, restaurants, shopping malls, or—and this is most important—airplanes. (The two places you are most likely to "pick something up" are an airplane or—as you may have guessed—a hospital.)

So there you have it: By caring for the strokee, you're getting as much benefit or more than you're giving and part of that benefit may well be a longer life and a freedom from communicable diseases.

THE RELUCTANT STROKEE

One of the greatest sources of frustration, sorrow, and even anger for a concerned caregiver is a mystery you might call "The Case of the Reluctant Strokee." I prowl the Internet for new developments in post-stroke therapy, read every magazine article on stroke that is published, and I get ideas—lots of ideas—for getting the strokee back into the mainstream of life.

In everything I read, it seems that the protagonist is always out there fighting valiantly every minute of every day for recovery. I can't understand when June doesn't follow this pattern. Doesn't she want to get better? If I were in her position I'd do everything humanly possible—and then some—to improve.

Or would I?

You never know if you're not the person involved. You can't know how much the therapy hurts and how much stroke fatigue you'd have. You can't know how discouraging it is when therapy after therapy, each of which promises great results, delivers nothing but disappointment.

I admit that in my quest there is more than a modicum of selfishness. I want June to get better as much for the freedom it will give me as it will give her. When she flatly refuses to try a new therapy or therapist I've discovered, or gives up—prematurely to my mind—on an old one that still has possibilities, it drives me crazy.

What drives *her* crazy is what I call "making suggestions" and what she considers "nagging" (translation: making the same suggestion more than once), "bossing her around" or "meddling."

June sums up the situation this way: "You're not running my therapies, I am."

I generally don't give up easily. Back when June was suffering chronic headaches I dragged her to doctors and clinics for five years until we found one who analyzed her problem and took care of it. But in this case I have had to finally capitulate. It just causes too much animosity between us—not a salubrious state of affairs. What finally pushed me over the line was talking to Dr. Richard Rubin, the psychologist with whom we collaborated on *Psyching Out Diabetes*. He is of the very sound opinion that "You can't make anyone do anything he doesn't want to do." Remember that when dealing with your strokee.

Dr. Rubin is right, of course. If you try to force the issue, all you'll get is a headache from the stone wall you're beating your head against. Your only hope lies in another Dr. Rubin quote: "People will only change when there's a real and very personal payoff for changing." Only if the strokee finds that real and personal payoff for him or herself do you have a chance. We'll see. As the philosopher Mort Sahl said, "The future lies ahead."

FOCUSING YOUR LIFE

You may have read the tragic story of the University of California at Irvine professor who was supposed to be driving his infant son to the university's day care center but, forgetting that the baby was in the car, he instead continued on to the parking lot. There he parked in his assigned place and went in to work, leaving the child to die of heat stroke in the car.

Ellen Langer, professor of psychology at Harvard University and author of *The Power of Mindful Learning*, asks "What was this man thinking?" and goes on to answer her own question, "Probably nothing." She calls this an example of "mindlessness."

As the headline of an article she wrote for the *Los Angeles Times* admonishes: "Be Aware of Life's Minefields; When we go through the day on automatic pilot, we risk tragedy." I'm sure I'm as mindless as the next person—or more so—and so probably are you. But as caregivers, I think our problem is a little different. You might call it "mind-too-fullness." You have too much on your mind and are trying to do too many things at the same time. Multitasking, thy name is caregiver.

A column by Sue Shellenbarger in the *Wall Street Journal*[15] bluntly points out that "Multitasking Makes You Stupid: Studies Show Pitfalls of Doing Too Much at Once." I don't need those studies to tell me that. I've lived it.

In the years I've been a caregiver, I've done many stupid things I never used to do, and I don't think it's a sudden onset of senility. For example, I find myself repeatedly incorrectly dialing familiar phone numbers. Sometimes I do this two or three times in a row. Once I was suffering a painful attack of "wheelchair back," a condition that caregivers get from lifting and pushing wheelchairs. In desperation I called a masseuse whom I use for emergency situations. I got her answering machine and left a message along with my number. Only it wasn't exactly my number, since I had transposed it as I found out when I called again after not hearing from her.

I've burned up two pans simply by forgetting to watch them or not putting on the timer to remind myself they were on the stove. One day I was taking a bath and heard three loud explosions. *Ka-bang! Ka-boom! Ka-bang!* I had no idea what was going on. A terrorist attack? No. I had left three eggs on the stove, they boiled dry and *Ka-Bang! Ka-Boom! Ka-Bang!* Bits of eggs and shell all over the kitchen.

Why do I do these things? A friend of mine chided me saying,

[15] *The Wall Street Journal,* March 27, 2003.

"You're not focused! You've got to get focused!" Well, yes, I know it. And you must know it if your brain seems unable to think and remember as once it did, and if, no matter what your age, you keep having the dreaded "senior moments." In that case we have no choice: Focus we must lest we court disaster of the caliber of the professor's.

BRAIN TRAINING

Chronic stress is the enemy of memory.
—GARY SMALL, M.D., DIRECTOR OF THE UCLA
CENTER ON AGING, *The Memory Bible*

Caregivers—especially this one—have a strong tendency to experience those "senior moments" when they go into a room only to find themselves standing there in confusion not knowing why they came in. You forget names of old friends and the location of places you have visited innumerable times and the titles of books you want to recommend. This could be blamed on stress—having too much on your mind and trying to do too many things at once. But no matter what causes it, it would be a good thing to get rid of.

In spring of 2003, the *Wall Street Journal*[16] ran an article called "Lobes of Steel: Giving Your Memory a Workout," which gave tips on boosting your memory, one of which was the old "use it or lose it" theory. The article suggested exercising your mind by playing bridge, learning a foreign language, doing crossword puzzles, and so on. This last suggested activity, crossword puzzles, was what Chief Justice Oliver Wendell Holmes used to keep his wits sharp until his demise at age ninety-four. But what fascinated me was the list of eight strategies for keeping the mind sharp (see page 158).

An amazing thing about June is that, despite her stroke, she

---

[16] *The Wall Street Journal,* April 29, 2003.

Eight Strategies for Keeping the Mind Sharp (adapted from the *Wall Street Journal*)

1. Eat berries (especially blueberries).
2. Eat foods rich in vitamin E (olive oil, spinach, and whole grains).
3. Get rid of stress.
4. Exercise!
5. Get enough sleep—tough especially if you have the night shift (on top of the day shift).
6. Ditch your calculator—engaging the mind in problem-solving of this sort can thwart memory loss.
7. Take on random mental problems. This idea was based on the fact that "mice in cages packed with stimulating toys demonstrated better memories than those in barren cages." One random task would be trying to reset the VCR clock yourself. Another thing you can do is listen to National Public Radio's *Sunday Weekend* edition. The "Puzzle Master," Will Shortz, has a session every week in which you can test your wits against the audience member appearing on the show. Then you can try to solve the weekly puzzle to see if you can be chosen for the following week's program. The puzzles are varied and challenging and will give your brain cells a good workout.
8. Try writing, eating, or using a computer mouse with the hand you don't normally use for such activities. This, to my mind, is the most significant and beneficial strategy for caregivers and strokees alike to stimulate hand-brain coordination and engage both lobes of the brain. I did this with my computer mouse but, unfortunately, after a couple of months I got as good with my left hand as with my right so I'm not sure I'm stimulating my hand-brain coordination. Maybe I should try using my feet.

has a very good memory—better, it seems, than before her stroke. Although she's ten years older than I, her memory is at least ten times better. I rely on her to remind me of things I need to do. Strategy 8 may have something to do with it. She must be firing on both cylinders, whereas I'm probably fumbling along with only one.

This has inspired me to bring my left hand to the party. I'm doing this for more reasons than one. First, it gives my right arm (and shoulder and hand) a rest. As a result of lifting June in and out of bed, in and out of the wheelchair, I've developed a number of pain points in my right arm and shoulder. Switching arms will help alleviate the pain. It also shows me how difficult it is to change physical habits later in life and causes me to develop a little more compassion and understanding for those who've had to make do as a result of a stroke or other disability.

Finally, if, through some accident of life, I become unable to use my right side, I'll have trained for it. The funny thing is that when I was working at Valley College library and was just embarking on a writing career, it occurred to me that if for some reason I couldn't write with my dominant right hand, I'd be in "a fine mess," as comedians Laurel and Hardy used to put it. So I decided to write book-order cards with my left hand. This went on for a few weeks, until by popular demand from those who had to read the cards I was forbidden to continue this practice. I now think that it's a pity I had to give it up. Otherwise I'd be totally ambidextrous by now. And even more's the pity that June, who was the head librarian at the time, hadn't recognized this for the brilliant idea that it was and decided to take it up herself!

SWEEPING THE MIND WITH MEDITATION

Meditation comes out of Eastern mystical tradition. We're concerned here not with the complex, centuries-old religious teachings of Buddhism associated with meditation, but with meditation as a relaxation and calming technique—just what a caregiver needs (in case you haven't noticed). It's our impression that some people may shy away from meditation because of its religious associations. But to quote Eknath Easwaran, author of *The Mantram Handbook,* "Meditation is not a religion; it is a technique which enables us to realize for ourselves the unity of life within any of the world's great religious traditions, or even if we profess no religion at all."

Meditation sweeps away your frets and fears and fatigue and releases you from the tyranny of that restless voice inside your head that never lets up on you except when you're asleep or un-conscious—your "monkey mind." Thubten Chodron, author of *Taming the Monkey Mind,* describes this simian sensibility thusly: "One of my teachers often compared our minds to monkeys: just as monkeys play with an object for a few moments and leave it in boredom and dissatisfaction to look for another thing to amuse them, so too do we run from thought to thought, emotion to emotion, place to place" and from task to task. (Caregivers are particularly susceptible to monkey mindedness.)

What is particularly good about meditation is that if you carry it off, it gives you a wonderful respite from those problems and worries associated with caregiving that are in your thoughts all your waking hours. If you practice it consistently, meditation can change not just your physiology but your entire life.

Busy Doing Nothing

The objective in all meditation is to control the attention. What you do is block out the chaos of the outer world and submerge yourself in your own peaceful inner world. Each school of Bud-dhism, each branch of each school, even each yoga or Zen master, seems to have a particular set of instructions for how to do this. Transcendental meditation (TM) is the meditative technique most of us have heard about, because it's been well publicized and advertised in the United States by its founder, Maharishi Mahesh Yogi. In TM, you restrict your attention by repeating a sound (mantra) over and over again while sitting with your eyes closed. TM is based on an East Indian form of Buddhism. In Zen, the Japanese form of Buddhism, you open up your attention by concentrating on your breathing.

We're going to discuss here only the beginning exercises for each of these two types of meditation. What we tell you may sound simplistic, but believe me, only the explanation is simplistic. The process itself is extremely elusive and takes dedication to master. Until you've tried it, you can't realize how almost utterly impossible it is to harness your mind or turn it off for even a few seconds, let alone for half an hour. (Ultimately you *can* do it, however.) Nor can you realize what a stunning relief it is from your normal state of awareness when you finally manage to do it, even briefly. I know your time is limited: Start with a few minutes or even seconds and see what happens.

Where and When to Meditate

Meditation should always be practiced in the same place, a place where you will not be interrupted and where there is no noise. Finding this serene atmosphere is often the biggest challenge.

There are numerous traditional positions for meditation. The classic is full lotus. To do this, you sit on a small cushion on the floor, placing your right foot on your left thigh and your left foot on your right thigh. But half lotus (right foot on your left thigh or vice versa) and even just sitting on the edge of a chair are perfectly acceptable for beginners and for those who don't want to risk cutting off their circulation. Select the position that suits you best. If it's not too cold, purists suggest doing your meditation in bare feet. Removing your wristwatch is also recommended. If you can fit it in, it's a good practice to meditate at the same time each day, and you can look forward to this time as a time free from stress. Early morning on arising and before breakfast is the best time for most people (meditating after eating is not recommended). Before dinner is a good time, too, but before going to bed is not, as it may heighten your consciousness so much that you can't get to sleep.

Start with five minutes a day and gradually extend the time until you can handle as much as half an hour. A short meditation done daily is far preferable to a longer one done erratically. And if you have to change time or place occasionally, do so rather than eliminating that day's practice entirely. You need regular practice to create that oasis in your daily life where stress dare not visit you.

Transcendental Meditation

Let's begin with transcendental meditation (mantra or sound) and then go on to Zen (breathing). The first step is to choose your sound. The mantra is usually short, as short as a single syllable or two, and should have a melodious sound. The TM'ers say it should have no special significance, but in much Hindu yoga practice the mantra is often an inspirational passage of several syllables or even words. Patricia Carrington, a Princeton University psychologist who uses meditation for mental therapy in her counseling practice, suggests that students in her program pick whichever of the following mantras sounds to them most pleasant and soothing: *ah-nam, shi-rim,* or *ra-mah.*

Diana Guthrie, Ph.D., CDE, suggests choosing a scripture to meditate upon. She uses "Be still, and know that I am God" (Psalms 46:10). Each time, as she repeats this verse, she makes it a shorter and shorter mantra by gradually eliminating words until she is down to the two words "Be still" and finally just "Be."

To do your mantra meditation, go to your chosen spot and take your chosen position. Take a few slow, deep breaths to quiet yourself, but not so deep that you become light-headed. Then close your eyes and start repeating your mantra slowly to yourself over and over again, breathing abdominally through your nose. As extraneous thoughts and images crowd into your mind, just let them flow through without allowing them to distract you from concentrating on your mantra. (When you are in this state, you cannot concentrate on any aspect of your caregiving.)

Meditating is something like placing yourself in an isolation chamber. And like other de-stressing techniques, it's virtually impossible to explain how to do it. In fact, some Indian teachers say that you don't "do" it. You create in yourself a state of non-doing and meditation happens spontaneously.

When you finish, stop repeating the mantra and sit, with your eyes still closed, for several more minutes. Rather than snapping yourself out of your meditative state, open your eyes, stretch the way you would when awakening from a nap, and then get up and resume your normal activities. You will feel refreshed and energized.

Zen Meditation

Turning now to the Zen technique, how you sit is very important. Use the full- or half-lotus position, or sit on the forward part of a straight chair. Your spine should be straight, the small of your back concave (abdomen pushed out) and your chin pulled in. Keep your hands in your lap, turned up, with the left hand inside the right, unless you're left-handed; in that case, the right hand should be inside the left. Your thumbs should be lightly touching. Keep your eyes open, looking about three feet in front of you and downward, but unfocused. Begin by moving your torso in a wide circle, gradually narrowing the circle until you come to a stop at your natural center, where you will feel balanced and secure.

Now sit there and let your mind follow the movement of your breathing.

Use abdominal breathing: in and out, in and out. Let other thoughts and images come but also let them go as you continue concentrating on your breathing. You can count one as you exhale if this helps, or one as you inhale and two as you exhale. You can even count your breathing all the way to ten, but no higher, as it would be distracting. Eventually you will get to the point where you can sit and feel your breathing without counting. In fact, Zen teachers (roshis) refer to Zen practice as "just sitting."

Medi-Teachers

Many meditators feel that for any form of meditation you should work under the direction of a teacher, because you need someone to answer your questions and help you with uncomfortable emotional and physical side effects that may appear as you are becoming de-stressed. But this is probably unrealistic for someone with your caregiver responsibilities. But if, perchance, you can carve out a regular chunk of time, one way to find a teacher is to check with community and four-year colleges in your vicinity. Many offer courses in meditation, and sometimes classes are held at the headquarters of yoga or Zen training centers. Meditation sessions with a religious emphasis are offered by some churches. You can find announcements about these in your local newspaper.

CAREGIVER WEIGHT GAIN

Yes, alas, we caregivers are very likely to put on weight. I have a friend who was caring for her mother, a thin wraith who was getting more so by the day. She had no appetite and virtually refused to eat. My friend had to sit there to match her bite for bite—and then some—or she wouldn't eat at all. My friend was literally eating for two and it showed in her weight gain. Examining the reasons why can pave the way for changing the behavior:

• We deserve a reward for all the work we do, for all the sacrifices we make. That nobody can deny! And what better and more accessible reward is there than food? We long for a tasty treat. And when we hear the siren call of the ice cream, the chocolate, the doughnut, or, as in my case the pistachio nuts, we answer it.

• We feel sad at our situation and that of the person we care for. We need to fill that empty feeling in the pit of our stomachs. With what do we use to try to fill empty feelings? You guessed it—food! (P.S. It doesn't work for more than a few moments.)

• We're nervous and upset. We wander toward a snack and unconsciously toss it down. Before long, almost having forgotten we ate something, we do it again . . . and again.

• We're bored. Each day is like the day before and the day before that and the day after and the day after that. We need to nibble on something to break the monotony.

• We do the cooking, and whatever the cook wants, the cook gets. When your favorite dishes are there before you on the table, and it may be the only good thing that happens to you today, the temptation to overeat is excruciating. You succumb to it.

• We're the ones to clean up after a meal. When there are leftovers, we have two choices. If there's enough for another meal, stow it in the refrigerator for later use. If there's *not* enough, throw it out immediately. Don't feel guilty that you're wasting food while children are starving in whatever land. If you eat it, it won't help the children and it will harm you.

• We are in a very uncomfortable life situation and it makes us long for comfort, especially comfort food—mashed potatoes and gravy, fried chicken, macaroni and cheese, custards, all kinds of soft and creamy things, whatever reminds us of our childhood when we were cared for and cosseted. Comfort foods are definitely not diet foods.

• Many of us have to get up a couple or three times a night to check on or help our patient. As long as we're up and awake we gravitate toward the refrigerator. There's always something in it.

Losing the Pounds

Just as, according to Paul Simon, there are fifty ways to leave your lover, there must be a hundred and fifty ways to put on caregiver pounds. Would that there were as many to get rid of them. But there are at least a few that I can offer you.

When it comes to the food that is irresistible to you, just don't keep it in the house. For example, as I mentioned, pistachio nuts are hard enough for me to resist, but a local market chain has pushed them over the line with chili-lemon pistachio nuts. After snacking up a whole bag in two days and another in another two days, I put them on my personal forbidden list.

You could have someone hide the forbidden irresistible and ration it out to you—but I doubt that would work. In a fit of unrequited desire, you might wind up ransacking the house the way the characters in the movie *The Days of Wine and Roses* tore up the greenhouse looking for a hidden bottle.

You could have that special reward comforting food at *one* meal, *once* a week.

You could make it a rule to never eat between meals. That's when the unconscious snacking takes place. Especially never eat anything between dinner and breakfast.

No second helpings, ever, and just a normal-size first one. It shouldn't be like a cartoon I once saw, which showed an exceedingly happy-looking man holding a martini glass that was about the size of a washbasin. The caption read, "Joe's doctor said he should limit himself to one drink a day."

This takes a bit of calculating, but if you do it and stick to it, it definitely works. Go onto a low-carbohydrate diet—and I mean *low*. Eat only 12 grams of carbohydrate per meal. For the other foods (fats and proteins), you can eat all you want so you don't feel starved and deprived as you do on more conventional diets. I can personally testify that this diet really works. The pounds just melt away.

Fortunately, now all packaged and processed foods must by law have the serving size and nutritional analysis on the package, making it very easy to figure your carbohydrate allotment. For all the other foods that don't come in packages, since the low-carb diet is so in vogue, you can find their analyses in one of the many carbohydrate guides available. For example:

- *Dr. Atkins' New Carbohydrate Gram Counter* by Robert C. Atkins
- *Complete Guide to Carb Counting* by Hope S. Warshaw
- *The Carbohydrate Addict's Gram Counter* by Richard F. Heller and Rachael F. Heller

There are also cookbooks galore if you really want to get serious about low carbing. Two of the best are by Fran McCullough: *The Low-Carb Cookbook* and *Living Low-Carb*.

Warning: Don't go onto a low-fat diet for weight control. It just doesn't work and will only leave you disappointed and frustrated. You have enough disappointments and frustrations in your life right now without adding more.

But there is one thing that works better than anything else and works well in conjunction with other dieting schemes. That is the wonderful wonder drug of exercise.

Some Things Caregivers Don't Get Enough Of: Exercise

In magazine and newspaper articles encouraging people to exercise more, they frequently say something like, "All you need to do to stay in good shape and in good health is exercise moderately for about thirty minutes a day."

"Hey, I can do that!" you say, as I said. But now the advice has changed. They're upping the ante to one hour a day. This actually makes more sense, but it does take up more time in a time-poor caregiver's life. I try to fit that much exercise in with a half hour of stretching and a half hour of walking, but I don't always succeed. And you shouldn't excoriate yourself if you don't either. Here are some tips on exercises that will be of most help to a caregiver. You should choose the one or ones that most appeal to you because you'll never keep doing exercise you don't enjoy. (It's hard enough to keep doing exercise you *do* enjoy!)

Walking

Walking is the best possible exercise.

—THOMAS JEFFERSON

Walking is the one sport that virtually anyone can do without risk. In fact, as one doctor put it, "It's impossible to walk too much." Here's the definitive endorsement of walking and other non-grueling physical activities. A study of 17,000 Harvard alumni revealed that you don't need to do arduous sports like running marathons to reap the lifesaving benefits of exercise. Men who pursued such moderate activities as walking, climbing stairs, and sports that used 2,000 or more calories a week had death rates one-quarter to one-third lower than their more sedentary fellow graduates.

Of course during the day, and probably part of the night, you spend a lot of time on your feet. If you added it all up, it would be a decent walk. But that's not as beneficial as taking a walk when you can be outdoors breathing the air and looking at flowers and trees and other people. But be it indoors or out, go for a walk whenever and wherever you can.

Of course, the exigencies of your caregiving role may not allow you to be out of the house trotting around the neighborhood for extended periods, so you have to keep moving around the house as much as possible, using stairs if stairs there be.

Bicycling

If you don't have the freedom to go for a walk, it's even more unlikely that you could get out for a real bike ride. But one thing you might do to keep the body in healthy motion is to invest in an Exercycle. Actually, it doesn't have to be much of an investment since people are always buying them, thinking having one around the house will inspire them to use it. It usually doesn't work that way, so the Exercycle winds up in a garage sale or advertised in the *Pennysaver* or *Recycler* (!) or whatever your local free advertising paper is called. Sometimes if people are really anxious to get rid of it, they will even give it away. If you mention to friends that you're interested in an Exercycle, one of them just might say, "Here, take the @#$%^& thing away. All I do is hang clothes on it. It's just in the way."

If the Exercycle is right there staring you in the face you just might get into the habit of hopping on it when you have a few spare moments—a healthy and stress-reducing habit to get into. To keep it from being boring—the death of any exercise program—watch TV or read as you pedal.

STRETCHING

Prevention and Relief for "Wheelchair Back"

If the strokee you care for is in a wheelchair full or part time, you run the risk of getting lower back pain from lifting the strokee in and out of the wheelchair or going up and down steps in a wheelchair or lifting the back wheels of the wheelchair to go around corners (a maneuver you should avoid). Even if the strokee doesn't use a wheelchair, there may be a lot of lifting involved in your caregiver duties, and stretching will help you get more flexible and keep back problems from developing.

The best and most popular book on stretching is the succinctly titled *Stretching* by Bob Anderson. Along with the basic stretching exercises of previous editions, the new (twentieth) edition includes stretching routines to do while you watch TV (caregivers have to fit in exercises when and where they can), before and after gardening, while traveling, etc. There are even stretching exercises for people in wheelchairs, which you can teach your strokee, and the two of you can work out together. The accompanying line drawings make the exercises easy to follow.

Back Pain Remedies for Dummies by back pain specialist Michael S. Sinel, M.D., and clinical health psychologist William W. Deardorff, Ph.D., is more for people who have a chronic back pain—or incipient chronic back pain. Accessible and comprehensive, covering both traditional and holistic approaches, the book contains many tips on how to reduce your back pain and prevent recurrences.

BEYOND STRETCHING

Yoga

A caregiver of any age and in virtually any physical condition can benefit from yoga exercises. They are not jarring to the body and you are never supposed to strain yourself to achieve a position. Gradual, gentle, nonpainful stretching is the order of the day. Many people find it hard to believe that yoga exercises produce the wonderful effects they do, because they never leave you feeling exhausted and sore the way many people think exercises are supposed to. We like yoga exercises for a dual set of reasons. First, they keep muscles and joints flexible, improve circulation, and free metabolism to work better. Second, they reduce mental as well as physical tension—a great need for caregivers. They do this by making you slow down, because the positions are meant to be held for a certain number of counts rather than done in fast repetitions like some types of body-conditioning exercises. Also, yoga instructors (we should say hatha yoga, as that's the official term for the physical aspect of yoga) usually also teach deep-breathing techniques. (Fast, shallow breathing is a sign of body stress.)

When doing yoga exercises, try to develop a sense of body awareness. As yoga instructors advise, turn off your ordinary mind, the one that's forever churning like a washing machine, and really get into the stretch. Move slowly, smoothly into the stretch. *Be* the stretch. Experience it mentally as well as physically. As you breathe, feel you are actually breathing into the muscle you are stretching.

If you can be released from duty for an hour or so you may want to sign up for a yoga course at your local community college or recreation department. Taking a course has the additional advantage of getting you out into the world and providing some social interaction with your classmates and instructor. You can

Books for Yoga

- *Back Care Basics: A Doctor's Gentle Yoga Program for Back and Neck Pain Relief* by Mary Pullig Schatz (Rodmell Press, 1992): This book deals with neck and back pain and provides an introduction to yoga. The gentle approach is particularly effective for people who are already in pain.

- *The New Yoga for People Over 50: A Comprehensive Guide for Midlife and Older Beginners* by Suza Francina (HCI, 1997): Since many caregivers fit into this age category—or if you're not in number but in spirit, after a period in the caregiving trenches—this book is for you. The yoga people say you are as old as your spine so this book can rejuvenate and revitalize you. The book is realistic and inspiring and helps guide you through emotional as well as physical problems.

- *The Woman's Book of Yoga and Health: A Lifelong Guide to Wellness* by Linda Sparrowe and Patricia Walden (Shambhala, 2002): Just as the majority of caregivers are in their mature years, they are also predominantly women. This book, by the former editor of *Yoga Journal* and a nationally prominent yoga instructor not only teaches the basics of yoga, but addresses the special needs of women through all stages of their life. Exploring health issues such as pregnancy, menopause, eating disorders, back problems, stress, and depression, the book helps you relax and bring balance into your life with the help of yoga.

Videos for Yoga

- *AM/PM Yoga for Beginners* by Rodney Yee (Mr. AM) and Patricia Walden (Ms. PM) (Living Arts, 1998). This is a novel approach. Two different instructors give you an appropriate group of exercises. The a.m. one wakes you, takes away morning stiffness, and energizes you for the rigorous day ahead. The p.m. one relaxes you and winds you down from the manifold stresses of a caregiver's duties. The video provides very clear instructions on performing each movement. A plus is the beautiful setting in which the demonstrations are performed. The a.m. one is set on a beach on Maui at sunrise. The p.m. one is at sunset in Death Valley.

• *Basic Yoga Workout for Dummies* by Sara Ivanhoe (Anchor Bay Entertainment, 2000). This video teaches the "daily dozen" basic yoga postures in a relaxed and accessible way, emphasizing both breathing and motion. It is easy to follow Sara Ivanhoe's friendly, no-nonsense approach and explanations. You will gain an understanding of yoga so you can fit it in your daily life, and it will give you a leg up should you later decide to join a yoga class.

also check the program guide of the educational-television channel in your area to see if it carries a yoga class, as many do. Books and videos are great for yoga, especially if you're confined to the house, as many of us caregivers are. You can open a book or pop in a video and have a mini yoga session any time you have a spare moment or two.

SLEEP

Shakespeare wrote, "Sleep . . . knits up the raveled sleeve of care." Obviously, he wasn't a caregiver. If you're on the caregiving night shift as I am, and as most caregivers are, sleep only knits up to about the elbow before you must get up and do some caregiving: provide food or drink or medication (in June's case test blood sugar and, depending on the results, take the appropriate action), assist with a bathroom break, or do whatever the strokee needs.

Usually this interruption of sleeve-knitting occurs two or three times a night. It can often be like caring for an infant. That's why in our house we jocularly refer to it as "first feeding, second feeding, and third feeding." And, just as with an infant, if you aren't awakened for help, you wake yourself up, worrying that something untoward is going on, so you struggle out of bed to go check on things.

Once you're up and take care of the situation, the problem is to get back to sleep again. Not an easy assignment. I have a continuing problem that if I can't get back to sleep, I get bored and turn on the radio. If something interesting is on, I start listening to it, often until the next "feeding." This results in my having terminal grogginess all the next day. I'm working on breaking this debilitating habit with only intermittent success (it helps if the radio battery runs out). However, there are some little nutritional helpers available to you.

Melatonin

It goes without saying that no matter how in need of sleep you may be, you should never resort to sleeping pills while on caregiver duty. But I'll say it anyway: *Never resort to sleeping pills while on caregiver duty.* You always have to be on the *qui vive* to make sure that if a crisis occurs you won't be too knocked out to know it's happening and take the appropriate action. That said, we often long for a magic pill that will as, Hippocrates advises, "First do no harm" but will give us a few hours of blessed sleep. Well, have I got a pill for you! We learned about its merits from James W. Anderson, M.D., whom we know from our writings in diabetes. He devised the HCF (high carbohydrate and fiber diet) for diabetics and later brought the wonders of oat bran to public notice. His latest foray in innovation is his book *Dr. Anderson's Antioxidant Antiaging Health Program.* In this he introduced us to melatonin. Actually we had a nodding acquaintance with it from our travels when we used it to adjust our internal clocks to time zone changes.

But through his book we discovered that melatonin is just what the doctor ordered for sleep-deprived caregivers.

First off, you won't be drugging yourself, because melatonin is not a drug, but a natural hormone secreted by the pea-sized pineal (meaning pinecone-shaped) gland in the back of the brain. Darkness stimulates production of melatonin, so your melatonin level goes up at night, making you feel sleepy. As you age, your melatonin production diminishes. That's why older people often have insomnia. This can be corrected with melatonin supplements.

But whatever your age if you're on a sleep-interrupted schedule like mine, melatonin can give you a ticket for a quick trip back to the land of nod. Here's the way I use it. When I go to sleep at around 8 I take a 1-milligram tablet (I prefer the cherry-flavored kind). This causes me to sleep straight through until I get called for "the first feeding," usually around 11. When I return to bed I take an additional half tablet. After the "second feeding," at approximately 3, if I'm feeling sleepy I try to make it on autogenics (see following), but if I don't go to sleep fairly quickly, as I usually do, I'll take another half tablet. On this regimen I get *almost* enough sleep and I *usually* wake up in the morning in a nongroggy state. You will need to experiment to see if you need more or can get by with less, and asking the advice of your pharmacist or doctor is always a good bet.

Another nice thing about melatonin is that it is purported to deliver many more benefits than improved sleep. Some say it slows the aging process, is an antioxidant against heart disease and cancer, prevents the onset of Alzheimer's disease, relieves asthma, helps victims of migraines, epilepsy, autism, balding (?!), schizophrenia, and Parkinson's disease, prevents diabetes, Down syndrome, and sudden infant death syndrome. If it did only half of these things, it would truly be a miracle worker. Shucks, I'd be happy if it did none of them but assured me of a good night's sleep, as it currently seems to be doing.

Autogenic Training

This is the one thing that is almost a surefire way of getting me back to sleep. Autogenics—the word means "self-generating"— is a tension-relieving method that involves repeating short, self-hypnotic sentences to yourself in order to influence your body to relax, and when a caregiver relaxes, sleep usually follows.

First close your eyes, breathe deeply, and exhale slowly a few times to get general body relaxation, and then *slowly* repeat to yourself the following sentences. As you say each sentence, concentrate on that part of your body and feel it doing what you are telling it to do.

"My right hand is very heavy" is the first suggestion you give your body. Feelings of heaviness indicate relaxed muscles. You repeat this to yourself several times, sinking into the heaviness. Next you concentrate on creating feelings of warmth.

"My right hand is very warm." Feelings of warmth indicate that blood vessels have dilated (relaxed).

Next you move on to: "My left hand is very heavy" and "My left hand is very warm." Once both hands are heavy and warm, the body starts communicating this message to the rest of the body and you help out with repetitions of: "My right arm is very heavy" and "My right arm is very warm," working your way through feet and legs and even abdomen and buttocks.

When you've relaxed the whole body, finish off with, "My heartbeat is calm and regular" (repeat four times), followed by four-time repetitions of "My body breathes itself," "My abdomen is warm," and "My forehead is cool."

If this doesn't work to put you to sleep—and it usually will— do the whole routine over again. Incidentally, you don't have to use autogenics just to put yourself to sleep. It works wonderfully well to relax any time you need to get out from under stress. The more you do it, the better it works.

Don't get discouraged if you experience the slipping-back syndrome. That is, you may seem to deteriorate in your ability to respond to these self-commands, but with continued practice you will surge ahead again. You'll find that the more you do it, the better it works.

If you want to do some research to discover whether or not you're living with the handicap of a sleep deficit, you could start by reading Dr. William Dement's book *The Promise of Sleep: A Pioneer in Sleep Medicine Explores the Vital Connection Between Health and Happiness and a Good Night's Sleep.* In it, Dr. Dement teaches you how to "reclaim healthy sleep" in your own life. As one reviewer put it, "This book will put you to sleep—and that's a compliment."

You could also check into the Web site www.sleepquest.com. Dr. Dement is its chief scientific advisor and writes a column for it. Sleepquest will also help you link up with other sleep-related sites.

IT DOES COMPUTE

But you don't have to literally compute with it—a computer, that is. Every caregiver should have one for personal entertainment and edification, as well as staying in touch with family and friends by e-mail. The problem may be you don't have a computer (and don't want one) or you don't know how to use one, and you may be afraid to even try. You are, in other words, on the wrong side of the digital divide. It's not surprising that you're there, because a vast proportion of caregivers are older women—and guess which group has the smallest number of Internet users? Older women (those over sixty). Only 14 percent of them are nourished by the Internet umbilical cord. Contrast this to 80 percent of the general population.

In your caregiving situation you need the Internet more than anybody. It can deliver you from the feelings of isolation and loneliness that may sometimes engulf you. It can entertain you with movies, and it can educate you in areas you've long wanted to explore.

You can also make life better for your strokee if you can order things on line for him or her: clothing, special food, and so on. Above all you can find information and equipment that may make living with a stroke easier.

Don't let the expense of a computer stop you. Computers get cheaper every day and many people are giving away their old computers. You may have a friend who will not only be happy to give you a computer but show you how to use it. You will need an Internet connection either via a modem (a device that is connected to a phone line) or a cable. The former is less expensive, especially if you share an already-connected phone line but the latter is *much* faster and doesn't tie up a phone line.

Don't let that old devil fear of computers stop you, either. They are very easy to use and getting easier every day. Many public libraries have free classes and free computers to use. There is also a nonprofit organization called Seniornet, which has centers throughout the country for instruction of older people. Their locations are listed on their Web site, www.SeniorNet.org. Seniornet also offers free self-paced online tutorials. These contain, in four lessons, information about the Web, explanations about how information is collected and organized, and tips for how to find things on the Internet, plus a glossary in which you can look up a word you don't understand.

If all else fails, an hour or so with a computer guru is well worth the investment. He or she can set the computer up for you and give you a lesson. If you should have a computer problem later, it will be comforting to have someone you can call to solve it for you.

Tip: My favorite search engine is Google. With a search engine you can do amazing things, like entering the words "stroke fatigue." Google will then provide you with a list of articles on that topic. You click on the ones you're interested in and they will spring onto the screen.

Another tip: If you and your strokee enjoy movies—old and new—and past broadcasts of TV series, but you find it hard to get to the video rental stores to check them out, or, more to the point, to get them back in time, as a newly born Internet surfer, your problem will be solved. There is a rental service called Net-flix with a catalog of more than 10,000 films on DVD. You can go to their Web site, www.Netflix.com, send them a list of the films you want to see, and for a monthly fee ranging from $13.95 to $39.95, depending on the number of films you want to have at one time (maximum eight, lowest number four), they will be sent to you. You can keep the DVDs as long as you want—no late fees! There's even a postage-paid envelope in which to return them. It's like having your own private perpetual film festival and is the perfect service for strokees and caregivers who find it difficult to get to the cinema.

You may feel that since you've become a caregiver your world has shrunk to the size of a pea. A computer with an Internet connection will show you a new world of unimaginable magnitude. Make it yours!

READ IT, DON'T WEEP

When I was in college I knew a young man I considered a genius. It seemed to me that he had read every book ever published. When any topic came up in class or over coffee, he could converse knowledgeably and even entertainingly on it, peppering his speech with book references. How I envied him. As I got to know him better I learned the secret to his success. As a child he had been very weak and sickly. He couldn't play outdoors and had to have home schooling when it wasn't as common as it is now. Since he was pretty much confined to quarters he did nothing but read. His parents brought home tons of books from the library for him. And thus he passed his childhood and early adolescence. Gradually his health improved and he was able to go on to college, where he was just like everyone else, except for that book-stuffed brain of his.

Thanks to my healthy and heedless childhood, I knew I could never catch up to my college friend. Then June's stroke and my caregiver duties confined *me* to quarters, and I could read and read and read. You can, too. If you live in a large enough city and have that computer I advised you to get, you can order books online from the library and they will be delivered to your nearest branch. When you read a book review in the newspaper or hear about a book you think you'd like, just order and read. If a computerized service isn't available in your area, establish a relationship with the librarians in your nearest branch. They're friendly folk. I should know since I was one for twenty years.

You'll never run out of ideas for books if you get your hands on a copy of *Book List: Recommended Reading for Every Mood, Moment, and Reason* by Nancy Pearl, a Seattle librarian and director of the Washington Center for the Book. In this book, Ms. Pearl arranges her favorite books in 175 lively and intriguing categories (for example, "Bird Brains," "Elvis on My Mind," "Shrinks and Shrinkees," "Grit Lit," etc.). I particularly cherish her very unlibrarian-like advice: "Abandon any book you don't like after fifty pages."

Books you won't want to ever abandon are those of the charming and heart-warming *The No. 1 Ladies' Detective Agency* series by Alexander McCall Smith. Set in Botswana, they record the amiable adventures of Precious Ramotswe, whom one critic described as "a cross between Kinsey Millhone and Miss Marple." I won't tell you more lest I spoil the delights that await you.

So when you're getting cabin fever or you're bored and lonely for friends or feeling sad and sorry for yourself what with the unrelenting and often overwhelming caregiver duties, don't weep, read. To paraphrase both Emily Dickinson and John Bunyan,[17] "There is no frigate like a book to take you out of the slough of despond."

YOUR RIGHT TO A LIFE

In a religious discussion of "Is there a God?" I once heard it said that if there is a God, then expressing devotion to him/her every minute of every day and night of your life is not enough. (The atheist's corollary was "and if there isn't one, then even one second of veneration is too much.")

Well, there's no doubt that there *is* a strokee in your life. He or she is right there before your eyes every minute of every day and night of your life. And still it seems your endless hours of devotion aren't enough. The strokee often wants more and you want to give more. I once saw a sign in a Dublin watchmaker's window. "If it can't be done, it won't be done." Keep that in mind. You can't keep giving more and more of yourself to caregiving. It can't be done, it won't be done, and you must not feel guilty about it.

Just as patients deserve—and indeed need—a bill of rights, so do caregivers.

---

[17] John Bunyan (1628–1688) wrote *Pilgrim's Progress,* in which the pilgrim passed through the Slough of Despond, among other allegorical places.

A Caregiver's Bill of Rights

* I have the right to take care of myself. This is not an act of selfishness. It will give me the ability to take better care of my loved one.

* I have the right to seek help from others even though my loved one may object. I recognize the limits of my own endurance and strength.

* I have the right to maintain facets of my own life that do not include the person I care for just as I would if he or she were healthy. I know that I do everything that I reasonably can do for this person and I have the right to do some things just for myself.

* I have the right to get angry, be depressed, and express difficult feelings occasionally.

* I have the right to reject any attempt by my loved one (either conscious or unconscious) to manipulate me through guilt and/or depression.

* I have the right to receive considerations, affection, forgiveness, and acceptance for what I do for my loved one as I offer these attributes in return.

* I have the right to take pride in what I am accomplishing and to applaud the courage it has taken to meet the needs of my loved one.

* I have the right to protect my individuality and to make a life for myself that will sustain me in times when my loved one no longer needs my full-time help.

* I have the right to expect and demand that as new strides are made in finding resources to aid physically and mentally impaired older persons in our country, similar strides will be made toward aiding and supporting caregivers.

—— Author Unknown (but *definitely* not unappreciated!)

THE LAST RIGHT: THE RIGHT TO A RESPITE

Definitions of a respite include "break," "rest period," "breather," and "relief," among others; but the best definition is "the gift of time," the most precious of all gifts for a frazzled caregiver.

Doesn't this sound like exactly what you need—a weekend or a few days, or even a vacation of a couple of weeks to give you a chance to recharge emotionally so you will return better prepared to handle you day-to-day caregiving responsibilities? Mercifully, that need is being met by a growing number of organizations.

- *Nursing homes* for strokees who need full time nursing care.
- *Independent living facilities* for those who can still get around on their own and be responsible for taking their own medications, but whom you would not feel comfortable leaving totally alone.
- *Assisted living,* a care middle ground that is by far the respite most needed—and used. A stay at one of these facilities usually includes meals, housekeeping, bathing, dressing, delivering (or at least reminding) about medications. Often there are fun and games—entertainment programs, bingo, bridge, arts and crafts, shopping excursions for those up to them, and so on.

A particularly good feature of these respite care centers is that they give you and the strokee a chance to get acquainted with the facility and to see if the strokee would be happy going there full-time, should the need arise later on. (Fifty percent of those who go to one of these centers for respite care wind up as full-timers.)

Something you might be able to do is spend a night or two with your strokee at the facility so you can evaluate the place and see how he or she gets along there. This makes it a more comfortable transition. It's best to start out with a short stay rather than a couple of weeks right off the bat. This way it's not so disturbing to the strokee, who may feel deserted.

CHAPTER 7

The Business of Caregiving for a Strokee

During June's seizure-related hospital stay, everything had seemed to be under control. A nurse from intensive care was to come up and change the location of June's IV because the one she had was leaking. The reason the hospital staff wanted the intensive care nurse to take care of such a matter was that June has such thin skin and difficult-to-find veins that it takes an expert to get blood, insert IVs, and do other blood work.

Since it appeared that my presence wasn't needed, I accepted an invitation from some friends to go to dinner and a play. It was wonderful to go out again, just like the good old days of yore. But as I was driving home, I had a sudden apprehension that something untoward may have happened in my absence. When I checked my answering machine it turned out my apprehension was correct. I had two calls from the hospital asking me to call immediately because they needed to do a procedure and had to have permission from me before they could.

When I called I was heartily chewed out by the nurse because they had been trying to call me for hours. With June's thin skin and small veins, even the expert found it almost impossible to insert the IV, so they wanted to put in a triple lumen catheter. This they could use for the IV and for drawing blood for tests, including June's multiple blood sugars tests. This would be inserted in her neck or upper chest. When I asked how long it would be there, the nurse said "forever." This immediately put me in mind of when my mother's doctor told me she wasn't eating and he wanted my okay to put in a feeding tube. I gave permission since, in my ignorance, I thought they'd just stick in the tube, use it as long as necessary, and then, when she was back on her "feed," as we Midwesterners put it, they'd take it out again. Not so. A feeding tube is for a long time, if not forever.

When I challenged the nurse about her "forever" statement on the triple lumen catheter, she immediately backpedaled, explaining she only meant they'd just keep it in as long as she needed it and then take it out. I asked if I could give permission over the phone. She muttered to someone off camera and then said I could. She took this opportunity to harangue me about how a doctor had been there all ready to do the procedure earlier, but since they couldn't reach me, he had left and now it would be the weekend so the doctor would have to be on call. Consequently she didn't know when it could be done. She twisted the knife a little more by adding that as a temporary measure they were able to insert a catheter—in June's foot!—as a stopgap measure, but she didn't think it would last the night.

I didn't want to do something as misguided as inserting Mother's feeding tube, so I said I wanted to check with Deding's (our caregiver) sister, who is a head nurse at a local hospital, to see if this is a good idea. The nurse harrumphed a bit, but said okay. I called Deding—even though by now it was 11:30. She called her sister, who luckily happened to be on duty that night. Deding's sister thought it actually would be a good thing for June since they had such trouble inserting IVs, and this could also help with her diabetes therapy. I called back and gave the okay for the insertion of the triple lumen.

Because the nurse had laid such a guilt trip on me, I added the explanation that this was the first time in three years that I'd gone out to the theater and I guess I'd better never do *that* again. She immediately backpedaled again, saying, "Oh, no! You can't do that! You have to get out *sometime*."

The next morning when I went to see June, I was dismayed to find her in much worse shape than the day before when, eyes wide open, she had been talking and squeezing hands to show strength, etc. Now she was just lying there, eyes closed, mouth open, making rasping, gargling sounds with every breath The respiration therapist had just suctioned phlegm out of her chest—not that it seemed to have done much good. We couldn't figure why she had changed so much over night, unless it was the stress of their trying to insert the IV. Finally at around noon the doctor (young and arrogant), whom I had never seen before, arrived to perform the procedure. Chaos ensued: people running around, arms waving, spending about half an hour deciding if they could do it in the room or if they should send her to the ER or ICU. They finally decided to do it in the room and after another half hour the deed was done and the doctor stalked out without a word, probably on to more prestigious assignments.

It took June three days to return to normal. I couldn't help wondering if they had been able to reach me earlier that she might have been spared much of the discomfort and the medical setback. Ah, well, that's all "water over the bridge" as June would say in her quaint mixed metaphor way. But at least I learned a valuable lesson, which I pass on to you. You must always make sure the hospital or rehab center knows how to get in touch with you at all times, because if you're inaccessible, the rule of life is that's exactly when a crisis will strike.

Preparing a letter for the hospital, rehab center, or other medical facility is an excellent idea. The letter can be inserted in your strokee's chart and will provide doctors and nurses a way to contact you in case of emergency. The following is a letter that I gave to our medical experts to be inserted into June's chart. You can adapt it for your own use.

Important Information Concerning **(Insert Patient Name)**

To Whom It May Concern:

If you ever need to get in touch with **(insert your name and relationship, and reason that you should be the one contacted)**[18] *to ask questions or make decisions about* **(insert patient name),** *please do the following:*

1. Call **(insert your name)** *at* **(insert your phone number and cell phone number if you have one).** *If you reach an answering machine, leave a message, but don't stop there.*

2. Call **(insert the name of secondary caregiver or other responsible friend or relative who always knows where you are)** *at* **(insert phone number and cell phone number if such exists).** *If you don't reach someone at this number/these numbers, leave a message. This person always knows how to get in touch with me and will have me call you back promptly.*

Thank you for your help in this matter.

Name
Address
Phone number or numbers

[18] For example, mine was "who has power of attorney for June Biermann."

HOSPITALS AND HEALTH AND REHABILITATION CENTERS

After one of her strokes, because of Medicare and insurance con-
straints, June was about to be bounced from the hospital and its
therapy program. Her doctor, feeling she had need of more therapy, strongly recommended that she go to a "nursing facility,"
which was right in the neighborhood. "Nursing facility" sounded
like "rest home" or "assisted care living" or other euphemisms of
that ilk—the kind of place Eugene McCarthy, who, at age eighty-
seven was residing at the Georgetown Residence, described as "a
cruise ship on the River Styx."

June had long ago stated she wanted no part of such a living
arrangement. In fact she had made me faithfully promise I'd never
under any circumstance send her to one of those, whatever it was
called. Strangely enough, when my father had his stroke, after the
hospital therapy stay he was remanded to one such institution.
When June's doctor told me the address of the place she wanted
to send June, it turned out it was the exact same place my father
had been sent to. I still remembered what it was like. It was what
I would think of as a Civil War warehouse for the wounded. In
large rooms, patients were lined up in their beds like so much
cordwood. And, yes, there was the unmistakable aroma of a not-
too-clean hospital. My father looked at me pleadingly, saying, "I
never thought I would wind up in a place like this." That did it.
I immediately made arrangements for him to go home.

After my vivid description of the facility my father had been
in and June's doctor had recommended for her, June's doctor
looked puzzled.

"That doesn't seem like the place I'm talking about," she said.
"I really think you'd like it. They have cats and dogs and birds
there." Cats and dog and birds?! I thought it would be more like

rats and roaches and bedbugs. When the doctor urged me to just take a look at it, I asked if June would get therapy there, the doctor said, "Of course."

I knew June needed more therapy than she would be able to get at home, so I relented and went to look at the place. I was amazed at the transformation that had taken place. It had a spacious, well-lit reception area with a large cage filled with finches flitting and chirping about from nest to nest. The admissions counselor told me that the facility had long ago been sold to another company and had been totally upgraded two or three times. I had brief encounters with some of the animals and other birds. There were no private rooms available at the time, and the rooms were not exactly Four Seasons or Peninsula caliber, but they were adequate and clean and, after all, June was only going to be there until her therapy clicked in and she could come home again.

And so it came to pass that June was transported from the hospital to the rehab center. June settled in and began her therapy the following Monday. She found her therapists there to be as good or better than those at the hospital. And the animals, as someone said, "gave the place a human touch." I kept bringing to June's bed Chance (a gray and white tabby) and Angel, who, despite the name, is a big, fluffy white male with pink ears. Angel sometimes stealthily appeared in the night and June awoke to find him peacefully sleeping at the foot of her bed.

If your strokee needs to go for a stroke-recovery-period-cumtherapy and loves animals as June does (see "Fur-Covered Caregivers," page 28), you should check rehab centers in your community to see if any allow pets. Not all of them do, because some state laws didn't permit them. We can hope that those laws will change because creature comfort is very beneficial to those in therapy—and their caregivers!

PATIENT ADVOCACY IS JOB TWO

Just what you need—another job to contend with on top of basic caregiving. But the job of patient advocate rises to equal or greater importance when the strokee is in the hospital or rehabilitation center. You need to be on the scene almost as much as you are when you're caregiving at home. Not only does your presence keep the strokee from feeling lonely and isolated, but these days hospitals and rehab facilities are so understaffed and the employees so overworked they can't keep an eye on everything that's going on. You have to be an extra pair of eyes—and ears and often even hands—to make certain your strokee is getting the best care possible. If something doesn't look right, you should report the irregularity immediately. And you may have to report it more than once and follow up to make certain the problem is taken care of. You have to border on being a nag. In fact, sometimes you have to cross the border into nagdom. It's your responsibility. You never know when you'll be needed to solve a problem or get the hospital staff on the right track when they start to go astray.

Things to look out for include:

1. Is your stokee being given the correct medications and in the correct amounts and on the correct schedule? This means being familiar with the medications and scheduling yourself. You probably are if you've been handling the medicating at home (and you will be handling it again when you return home).

2. Is your strokee being kept clean, either with showers or sponge baths or a combination of the two?

3. Are the rooms and the corridors regularly—and thoroughly—cleaned?

4. If your strokee needs a special diet, is it being served for all

three meals? Does it allow some personal variations to avoid boredom and concomitant loss of appetite?

5. Is the facility quiet enough at night for your strokee to get a good night's sleep? You may have to make arrangements to stay there overnight to check this out for yourself.

6. Are they checking for bedsores carefully and often? (See page 119.)

Personhood

Another thing you should do as a patient advocate is to make sure your strokee is regarded as an individual, a human being with a personality and a past life and not just the anonymous "stroke victim in 16A." You can do this by getting to know the staff members personally and calling them by name in conversations. It's also important for you—and them—to always refer to the strokee by name.

One thing I did to personalize June to the staff was to put some past pictures of her on the corkboard in her room. One photograph was taken when she was the head librarian at Los Angeles Valley College. Another was with Eleanor Roosevelt, who, after she gave a talk at Valley College, was signing a book for the library's collection. I also put up pictures of June's Scottish Fold cats, Mary and Lucy. These photos made great get-acquainted conversation starters. If we found out that a staff member had a relative or friend with diabetes, we brought in a gift copy of one of our books on diabetes. It wasn't long before everyone in the place knew who June was and—equally important—*she* knew who *they* were. It made a warmer, happier situation for all concerned, including the caregiver.

June was so appreciative of the kindness and understanding given to her by the staff that on her birthday she provided a buffet lunch for them with Philippine cuisine arranged for by Deding. A good time was had by all.

KEEPING YOUR STROKEE FROM GOING DOWN THE TUBES: AN EXAMPLE OF PATIENT ADVOCACY

This harkens back to June's first stroke. At that time there was no doubt that she needed a gastrostomy (feeding tube through the stomach), since not only was she fairly *non compos mentis,* but she kept pulling out the nasogastric tube (feeding tube through the nose). When I voiced my fears of the tube being a permanent fixture in June's life to the gastroenterologist, he assured me that when she no longer needed it, he would take it right out.

After a few weeks, June was starting to eat "like a real person"—as she put it—and the tube became mere décor. I suggested that it be taken out. This they didn't want to do because they thought she might need it again. She never did, but despite my pleas the tube remained and continued to remain even after June had gone home and hadn't used the tube in weeks. I kept asking and asking for it to be removed. I admit that this was partially due to selfish reasons, because every few days I had the chore of flushing it out. But still the gastroenterologist who had put the thing in continued to refuse. I couldn't figure out why. One person on the staff told me that maybe they thought June might have another stroke, and it would be hard on her to have it reinserted. The gastroenterologist also countered my repeated requests with some kind of gobbledygook about how the tube had to stay in a certain length of time or else something bad, which he didn't elaborate upon, would happen. (Remember how he said he could "pull it right out" when it was no longer needed?) Finally, after about eight weeks of my incessant nagging, the doctor deigned to remove it. By that time I was so furious that I challenged him about why he had been so cruel as to keep her stuck with the tube all that time when it wasn't necessary. I'm happy to say this seemed to wound him deeply: I guess doctors are sensitive about accusations of cruelty.[19]

Given this background experience, it's understandable that when June was in the hospital for the seizure, there were mutterings that they wanted to insert a gastrostomy feeding tube. Actually it was more than mutterings: Three different doctors, one a gastroenterologist, announced they were going to do it and started making plans to schedule the procedure. Fortunately, while this was going on, the saint (as I now think of him) of a neurologist, when making his rounds, allowed as how June was getting a lot better. I took this opportunity to complain of the fact that they were trying to put a feeding tube in her, and that I was totally opposed to it. He looked puzzled and asked if they had done a swallowing test. "Not to my knowledge," I said. The holy man of medicine said he would order one. Strangely enough, the afternoon of this encounter, the gastroenterologist came in to announce that he would be inserting the tube the next morning. "Oh, no you won't! " I said with more firmness than I had ever used with a doctor. "Not until she has her swallowing test." He nervously backed out of the room, never to be seen or heard from again.

June passed the test with flying colors.

This is one reason why it's so important for the caregiver to be an assertive advocate for his or her strokee. So many caregivers are initially quiet as mice, thinking that the doctors must know best,

---

[19] I did additional research on the subject of gastrostomy tubes because I wanted to be sure there was no reason for keeping the thing in so long. Not only did nurses I asked about it confirm that the tube should have been taken out when June was eating normally, but I found the following on The Patient Education Web site, a resource center set up by the National University Hospital: "If you are able to eat orally and your doctor has approved this, it is encouraged to do so . . . The tube can be easily removed . . . The opening in the abdomen will close by itself quite easily." If I didn't know better I'd think the doctor was being paid by the number of days he kept the wretched thing in.

and if the information they're offering is confusing, well, then that's just the caregiver's fault for not understanding. Nonsense. You have every right—and, for your strokee, every obligation—to speak up.

In the case of the feeding tube, without my insistent intercession (some would call it intermeddling), June would have become the woman with *three* navels: one she was born with, one from the gastrostomy tube she had after her first stroke, and this ill-considered, ill-conceived one.

SOME FINANCIAL CONSIDERATIONS

As caregiver, you may be faced with some tough financial dilemmas due to your strokee's disability. As mentioned, some strokes are mild enough that the strokee can get back to work, and fairly quickly. Other strokes are so debilitating that the strokee must quit his or her job and stay home full time to recover. That means, of course, that as caregiver, you must also be around to help the strokee get through rehabilitation. The Family Caregiver Alliance estimates that the cost to businesses who lose female employees to caregiving alone is estimated at $3.3 billion. What this translates into for many caregivers is a loss of salary. A recent article in the *Detroit Free-Press* revealed that, according to a 1999 MetLife study, caregivers often pay out-of-pocket expenses averaging $19,525 while caregiving, not to mention lost wages and benefits, which can total a staggering $659,139 over their lifetimes.

Money may be tight, so look for ways to recoup some of your costs without cutting corners.

One thing you will most certainly have to begin doing, if you haven't gotten in the habit of doing this for your household expenditures, is budgeting. Take a long hard look at your budget and begin to itemize every anticipated expenditure related to caregiving: special equipment, food, hygienic products, medical expenses not covered by insurance (along with those therapies that are not covered), and so on.

Except for the occasional (and paltry) state tax break for caregivers (more on that below), the government doesn't help caregivers much when it comes to making ends meet. Some people erroneously believe that the federal government, in the form of Medicare, will cover some expenses for long-term health care. As we've seen, that simply isn't the case. And, as we've also seen, even your standard health insurance may be of no help at all.

The few things you can to do ameliorate the financial burden include knowing all you can about your strokee's disabilities and needs, so you can plan how much you may be expected to spend; seek information and guidance from support groups, friends who caregive, and even community organizations and your church, synagogue, or mosque.

Tax Credits

Some states offer caregivers tax breaks for long-term care. California, for instance, offers its citizens a modest tax break for long-term caregiving (about a $500 tax credit). Be sure to call your state tax office to discover whether or not your state offers something similar. In Washington, a few proposed bills giving caregivers a tax credit for caregiving have been introduced by presidents (notably Clinton) and various Congresspeople, but so far have not passed.

THINGS ARE LOOKING UP

The future belongs to those who prepare for it today.

—ATTRIBUTED TO MALCOLM X

Expect the worst and enjoy the best.

—IRISH SAYING

Homes of the Future

An article in the *Wall Street Journal* titled "The House of the Future—Yours"[20] by June Fletcher revealed that when it comes to planning ahead, some of us are more intelligent—and possibly prescient—than others of us. Able-bodied and people as young as their thirties are building homes designed to be what they call "elderly friendly" because they want it to be their "house for life no matter what may befall them or, perhaps their aging parents who might need to live with them." The needs of the elderly are almost identical to those of the handicapped of any age. For example:

- No "saddles" in doorways so a wheelchair can easily pass from one room to another.
- Extra-wide doors.
- Doors with leverlike handles instead of doorknobs.
- Grab bars. Since they can be obtrusive it is suggested that thick plywood could be placed behind the hall and bathroom walls so grab bars can be easily installed when the need arises. Since we had to retrofit grab bars, we discovered white grab bars, which are just as sturdy, but much less institutional-looking.
- Ramps leading to the front and/or back doors. This does a great deal toward keeping the strokee from feeling like a prisoner of disability.
- Front-loading washers and dryers for easier opening and loading.

There are also a number of big-ticket elder-and-handicapped-friendly items being introduced. These include:

- Motorized kitchen sink that can be raised to standard height or lowered for those in a wheelchair. (Approximately $900)

[20] February 14, 2003.

- Delta e-Flow faucet. This turns on and off electronically when you pass your hand under it. (As much as $500)
- Luxury Lift Home Elevator that fits in the space of a closet. It has an emergency lower system in case power should go off. ($30,000)

Of course, all these alterations are much less expensive if you install them as the house is being built rather than after the fact. And, costly though they may be, they do enhance the value of the house as demand is created because of the aging and possibly ailing Baby Boomers.

There is also the somewhat superstitious idea of "If you have it you probably won't need it and . . ." Well, you know the rest of the equation.

PAUL BERGER CONQUERS THE WORLD WITH AN ATTITUDE

An attitude not only of defense, but defiance.

—THOMAS GILLESPIE, *The Mountain Storm*

At age thirty-six, Paul E. Berger had a hemorrhagic stroke—a ruptured blood vessel in the brain—the same flavor as June's. The stroke left him with aphasia (an inability to speak), a paralysis on his right side that was like having a "permanently broken right arm and hand," and his right leg was not able to support him. The story of his road back is told vividly and movingly in his book *How to Conquer the World with One Hand . . . and an Attitude* (Positive Power Publishing, 2002). The part that will resonate most with strokees and their caregivers is the description of his therapies and—more importantly—the time it took to accomplish his improvements.

One thing that particularly infuriated Paul was the perpetuation of the old myth that "stroke survivors only benefit from short-term therapy." We'd been told this as well, even more specifically, that if the improvement didn't take place within six months, it wasn't going to happen. We kept waiting for the legendary six-month door to slam when we knew we'd have to give up and just resign ourselves to whatever condition June was at the time.

Fortunately for us and for the rest of the strokee community, Paul wasn't going to take this lying down, or in a wheelchair. When Nixon's "massive stroke" was announced in headlines (strokes always seem to be "massive" in newspaper write-ups), a neurologist explaining the situation said that had Nixon lived "He might have seen improvement for three to six months following the stroke." That did it for Paul. His fury was massive. It was so misleading to so many. Paul persuaded his wife, Stephanie, to write a letter to the editor to show his post-stroke progress and set the neurologist—and the readers—straight:

> *In two years, Paul had a vocabulary of about 100 words. In five years he could form simple sentences and had a vocabulary of about 1,000 words. In seven years he could form more complicated sentences and had regained many complex, multisyllabic words.*
>
> *By six months, he could stand and walk a few steps with another person's assistance. By nine months, he could stand and walk about with a cane; by two years, about six blocks with a cane. By five years, he could do a mile with a cane and a few rest stops. By seven years, he could walk a mile nonstop without a cane.*

The letter was published in the paper, and as the ripples spread out in the consciousness of the therapy world, a physical therapy magazine featured Paul and Stephanie, along with Paul's therapist in an article entitled "Long-Term Therapy Enables Stroke Victim to Regain Independence." Paul's goal was to prove to therapists and patients that the six-month rule was a vile—and destructive—

canard, and that strokees and their therapists shouldn't ever give up. Show them he did—in spades!

Times They Are a-Changing in Paul's Direction!

Fast forward four years, to April 7, 2003. An article by Jane E. Allen in the Health section of the *Los Angeles Times* appears with the headline: "Stroke therapy sets its sights higher, farther; Agility and strength can improve long after traditional rehab programs are through, researchers show." The article went on to show the inadequacy of the current six months of therapy, a wheelchair or a cane, and bye-bye.

"I don't think there is any hard limit on how long after a stroke people can continue to recover," says Michael Weinrich, director of the National Center for Medical Rehabilitation Research in Bethesda, Maryland. Others are starting to follow in line with this new belief, and approaches like "neuro-rehabilitation therapy" are coming to the fore. According to the article, this therapy "relies on drawing on the brain's ability to rebuild itself, to learn new tasks . . . neuroscientists and physical therapists are finding that repetitive, challenging and individualized therapy can rewire the brain and improve stroke patients' ability to move, put words together, and articulate them clearly—not just months after their attack, but even years later."

The new therapies include special treadmills with a supporting harness to retrain leg muscles, and the constraint-induced movement therapy (described on page 54). The big problem with these new therapies is the old familiar one of cost. It's not cheap (as much as $3,500 for sixty-five hours of constraint-induced therapy), but it's bound to get less expensive, as anything does, as its use increases. If insurers can be convinced of the benefits of the new therapies to them in terms of reduced costs of hospitalization, nursing and rehab facilities, falls, etc., then coverage of these therapies may be a reality.

One way the costs may be reduced in the future is by using robots to do the repetitive motions of the new therapies. (Look on the Internet under "Robots for Stroke Therapy" to see write-ups of some of the successful programs currently in operation.)

BETTER STROKE RECOVERY THROUGH CHEMISTRY

In conjunction with the new therapies, the *Los Angeles Times* reports that some stroke centers are starting to use medications that "bathe the brain in chemicals thought to enhance learning and brain function." For example, doctors at Duke University add the stimulant dextroamphetamine to the therapy mix in an attempt to improve mobility while researchers at the Rehabilitation Institute of Chicago, working to advance the progress of speech therapy, use bromocriptine (Parlodel), a medication previously used with Parkinson's disease patients.

As Dr. Mary Ellen Michel, program director for stroke and traumatic brain injury at the National Institute of Neurological Disorders and Stroke, says, "I don't think you give up on the brain." And we don't think you give up on the person carrying that brain around and putting forth the tremendous effort to bring it back to full life—especially if that person is your strokee.

CHAPTER 8

Other People's Strokes

Some of the best inspiration comes from hearing of others who have suffered strokes, but who have triumphed—overcoming aphasia or dysarthia, learning how to walk again, getting back into the swing of beloved social activities, and so on.

June feels a strong kinship for Katherine Sherwood even though she has never met her, never written or e-mailed her, never talked to her on the phone. Katherine is an artist and associate professor of art at the University of California, Berkeley, June's alma mater. They both suffered the same kind of stroke—hemorrhagic (bursting of blood vessels)—on the left side of the brain and both women came close to not surviving the event. The right sides of both June and Katherine's bodies have been impaired by the stroke. You've already read the story of June's stroke. Here is the rest of Katherine's story and its amazing denouement.

KATHERINE SHERWOOD:
PAINTING HERSELF OUT OF A CORNER

I never appreciated how therapeutic art could be until I went through this experience. This is by far the most effective occupational therapy I underwent.

—KATHERINE SHERWOOD

In May 1997, at the age of forty-four, Katherine was critiquing a graduate student's work when she was suddenly hit by an excruciating pain in the upper left side of her head. Within seconds her right side was paralyzed. She was rushed to the emergency room where she was diagnosed as having had the proverbial "massive stroke." She couldn't walk, speak, or use her right hand—the painting hand.

When she went home after six weeks in the hospital, her right side remained paralyzed. She could talk, but as an article on SFGate.com put it, she "had acquired a mysterious Blanche Dubois–like Southern accent that doctors suggested harkened back to early language memories from her New Orleans childhood." She could walk, but with difficulty; at first she had to use a cane. Without the cane she says, "It feels like I am having to carry around buckets of concrete on my right side." Katherine's daughter, Odette, who was four at the time of her mother's stroke, kept asking Katherine about when her "broken leg and arm" would get better.

As Katherine gradually came to realize the answer to that question was probably "never," she understandably grew depressed; but despite the dismal prognosis that the paralysis might be permanent, she continued to be determined to awaken the former skills of her painting hand and to rebuff those people who suggested that she try painting with the left.

Then it came to pass that she was in her radiologist's office having a carotid angiogram to see if there had been any further bleeding in her brain. In her sedated state when she saw the blood vessels of her brain displayed on the computer screen, it looked like a Chinese painting from the Sung dynasty, a period of art she particularly loved. When the session was over she asked for a copy of the angiogram. Although, as she said, "The technician thought I was crazy," he complied with her request.

She made prints out of the images and, "because I wanted to paint them, I had to use my left hand." Switching from oil to acrylics, she painted by laying the large canvases on an old bed frame and scooting around them on a wheeled office chair, feeling "strangely liberated." Once her left hand got into the picture it was there to stay, producing remarkable, no, make that amazing results. Her husband, artist Jeff Adams, said that her art "just flowed . . . She's making the paintings she always wanted to." She, herself, marvels at what comes out, saying, "I am frankly amazed that I am able to do these paintings . . . Sometimes I look at my work and ask, 'Did I paint that?' . . . It's almost as if the ideas just pass through me instead of originating in my head." The creative blocks that formerly plagued her have disappeared.

When Katherine exhibited some of her new left-handed paintings, it was clear that she had become a much better painter than she was in her right-handed days, eliciting such critical comments as "breathtaking," "raw," "intuitive."

Lawrence Rinder, a curator at the Whitney Museum of American Art says of her new paintings: "It's as if she pulled out all the stops. It is rare to see work that impressive, fresh, and powerful." Janet Bishop, a curator of the San Francisco Museum of Modern Art, echoes these sentiments. "The new work is more robust, visceral, and physical." San Francisco art critic Kenneth Baker says, "Her work has acquired an urgency that it didn't have before."

The art world, recognizing her as a rising star, has begun giv-ing her awards and putting its money where its praise is. Her pre-stroke paintings sold for around $7,000. Her canvases currently go for up to $20,000.

What has brought about this remarkable change in Katherine's paintings? San Francisco neurologists say that people who suffer damage to the left side of the brain sometimes experience new creative insight. Other neuroscientists believe that the hemor-rhage could have remapped the circuitry inside her head in a way that strengthened her more artistic right side.

But never mind the scientific whys and wherefores: The fact remains that Katherine Sherwood has survived her ordeal, is painting better than ever before, and is even back teaching her art classes to the delight of her students, one of whom, Christine Lyons, says, "She really challenges her students to question our work and to help us find our own voice." She calls Sherwood a consummate teacher and artist. "You know you're working with the real deal."

To learn more about Katherine Sherwood and her works, look up "Katherine Sherwood" on Google on the Internet. Of particular interest are her post-stroke paintings inspired by her angiograms.

Star Power

Luminaries of the entertainment industry often seem immune to the vicissitudes to which the rest of us mere mortals are subject. Their Technicolor, big screen lives as portrayed on TV and in the press glow with a mystical protective power. This seems especially true when you're struggling with post-stroke traumas while they merrily romp through their charmed lives. But it ain't necessarily so. Here are three examples of stars who suffered all the slings and arrows that other strokes experience, yet with luck and pluck and a fierce determination, emerged triumphant.

KIRK DOUGLAS: A CHAMPION GETS UP
OFF THE MAT WITH A RENEWED LUST FOR LIFE

Reading the opening pages of Kirk Douglas's *My Stroke of Luck,* we were impressed by the skill with which it was written. Wow!

I am an eighty-year-old man with a stroke. I'm an actor, and I can't talk. Is this THE END? Maybe I could study with Marcel Marceau and become a mime, but the thought didn't make me laugh . . . With an effort, I pulled myself out of bed and stumbled to the bathroom. I dared to look in the mirror. My tongue was thick. I couldn't swallow my saliva fast enough; it was constantly dripping out of the corner of my mouth, drooping on the right side. My face was grotesque. I could not stop crying. I felt such deep shame and disgust. I hated myself . . .

I walked over to the desk. In the lower drawer is the gun I used in *Gunfight at the O.K. Corral* . . . In another drawer, I had a box of bullets. I took out two of them, and with the other hand flipped open the chamber of the gun. I loaded the gun and looked at it. In my mouth or at the temple?

I stuck the long barrel of the gun in my mouth and it bumped against my teeth. "Ow!" It sent shivers though my teeth, and I pulled the gun out.

I began to laugh. A toothache delayed my death.

Looking back on his aborted suicide attempt he now says that "suicide is stupid and selfish." Armed with that knowledge and a sense of humor, as well as the tough-love support of Anne, his wife of fifty years, he battled back from depression to the point that he could speak at the 1996 Academy Awards Ceremony, at which he was awarded an Oscar for lifetime achievement.

At the 2002 Academy Awards he joined his son Michael in presenting the award for the best picture. His performance at this event elicited this letter to the editor in the *Los Angeles Times*.

At a time when we are witnessing acts of incredible bravery by young Americans in the Iraqi desert, we are privileged to have been witness to a far different act of grit and valor in, of all places, the Kodak Theatre. The hero: none other than Kirk Douglas.

When he made his way painfully across the stage to join his son Michael as an Oscar presenter, he was courage personified. When, striving against the ravages of a debilitating stroke that has affected his speech, he managed to caution Michael to "speak distinctly." That was effort above and beyond any call to duty. Though perhaps emotionally draining for stroke victims and their families to watch, it was proof beyond dispute that recovery is possible— perhaps not in the sense of being wholly restorative, but certainly in a measure many victims now believe beyond their grasp.

Since his stroke Douglas has also appeared in two films: *Diamonds,* with his old friend Lauren Bacall, and *It Runs in the Family,* featuring three generations of Douglases (Kirk, his son Michael, and Michael's son Cameron, along with Kirk's former wife, Diana).

Of course, the stroke brought changes to his life, surprisingly many for the better. According to his son, Michael, he has mellowed.

"He had much less patience before . . . He's more fuzzy and, truthfully, a much nicer person." He also said that his dad is a better golfer now because "he doesn't try to kill the ball."

Kirk, himself, believes his stroke changed him in ways that enriched his life.

"It has given me so much understanding that I have never had before. [It] changed me into a better person, a person whom I like. We all want happiness. I've learned we achieve happiness when we seek the happiness and well-being of others." While he was in the depths of depression, huddled in his bed and entertaining those thoughts of suicide, he had a personal epiphany.

"What ultimately got me out of bed was the realization that I was thinking too much about my own misfortune. Depression is so self-centered. I found that when I began to think about the well-being of others, I began to feel better."

He attacked thinking of other people with the vengeance of Spartacus. He wrote his stroke book to be what he called "An operator's manual to help others overcome adversity and battle back. " He dedicated the book to his colleagues Christopher Reeve and Michael J. Fox "because they've shared their misfortune with the public and they've tried to help other people. You owe that because in my profession we depend on the public so the least you can do is try to help them if you can."

He has also put his money where his heart is. He and his wife have given away millions to charitable causes both in this country and overseas. Their latest project is rebuilding all the Los Angeles School District playgrounds and exercise facilities, which were in deplorable condition after all the cuts in education financing. As of this writing the score is 170 done, 130 to go.

Douglas has established an Alzheimer's unit in the Motion Picture and Television Hospital. It's called "Harry's Haven," named after Douglas's father. The goal of the unit is to care for the industry members with dignity, compassion, and the most advanced therapies.

PATRICIA NEAL: A THOROUGHBRED WINS THE ROSES

When you call upon a thoroughbred, he gives you all the speed, strength of heart and sinew in him. When you call on a jackass, he kicks.

—PATRICIA NEAL

A goodly number of moons ago—way before stroke entered our picture—June and I were in New York, and, after a museum morning, were having lunch in a small Italian restaurant on West End Ave. Shortly after we sat down, in walked Patricia Neal. I vaguely remembered that she had had a stroke, but she seemed to be in good fettle. She was walking unassisted and certainly had no facial evidence of a stroke. She also seemed to be a regular at the restaurant because all the employees greeted her warmly. We didn't approach her because we don't like to bug celebrities—and at this time we had no particular interest in strokes. Of course if it happened now we would probably dump our reticence and jump on her like a duck on a June bug.

Later on, after June's stroke struck and we were researching this book, we were shocked to read "Patricia Neal, 39, last year's Oscar-winning best actress who copped five prizes for her first Broadway performance in 1947, died last night at UCLA Medical Center." Wait a minute. This does not compute. Since it was now 2003, if she won acting awards in 1947, she'd have to be a tad older than thirty-nine. Finally we calmed down and read on. It turned out this was a headline written in *Variety* in 1965. Instead of dying she fooled everyone by hanging in there through three strokes and twenty-one days' worth of coma. As she said, "I think I was born stubborn, that's all . . . There were many who didn't think I would pull through. I had to have an operation that lasted seven hours, and I know very well my doctor thought I would conk out in the middle of it; but as I told him later, we Tennessee hillbillies don't conk out that easy, so I stayed alive." Actually, she was staying alive for two: she was pregnant with Lucy Neal Dahl, who was born 160 days after her stroke. "My first reaction was my utter amazement," she said, "the blessing that she was perfect."

At the rehabilitation center where June went after having a seizure, there was a nursing assistant named Neima who was from

Morocco, where she was formerly a French teacher. June and I enjoyed practicing our French with her. One day Neima asked me how June was doing and I said with my best Gallic shrug, *"Comme ci, comme ça"* (so-so), and she replied *"haut et bas, haut et bas"* (up and down, up and down), as if it were one of the inevitables of stroke life—as it is. Nowhere was this phenomenon more evident than in Patricia Neal's life. And her *hauts* were as far up as a *haut* could go and her *bas* as far down.

She was born with nascent beauty and talent, which quickly emerged. Because of her obvious ability at performing in local church programs, at age twelve her parents gave her acting lessons for Christmas. These took so well that upon graduation from high school she enrolled in the drama department of Northwestern University. She left there after two years, but that was no *bas*. It was a definite *haut* because after joining her drama coach for summer theater, she headed for New York and still more *hauts*. In only a few months she got a job as understudy in *Voice of the Turtle*. After that she appeared in a summer theater production of *Devil Take the Whistler,* where she was discovered by Lillian Hellman, who cast her in *Another Part of the Forest,* for which she won five awards including a Tony and a Drama Critic's Award—at age nineteen!

Then it was on to Hollywood, where along with several inter-mittent—and hugely successful forays to Broadway—she made thirteen movies with some of the biggest male stars, including Gary Cooper, whom she called "the love of my life." But here a *bas* en-tered the picture because he was married and wouldn't ask his Catholic wife to give him a divorce, so in 1951 that was that. She describes this sorry situation in her book, *As I Am.*

In 1953 she married author Roald Dahl and they had their first three children: Olivia in 1954, Tessa in 1957, and Theo in 1960. Her career was flourishing and her personal life contented, then along came the inevitable *bas*. The babysitter was pushing four-

month-old Theo in his carriage. When she entered the street after
the traffic light changed, a cab turned the corner and hit the carriage, which was thrown into the side of a bus. Theo had multiple head injuries, which led to eight brain surgeries and three
years of treatments for the removal of excess fluids. And the *bas*
beat went on. In 1962, Neal's oldest daughter, Olivia, died from
measles encephalitis,

But, displaying her Seabiscuit-like thoroughbred courage, Neal
continued with her career, winning the best actress award in 1963
for her role in *Hud*. She also received the joyous news that she was
pregnant again. But this *haut* period was followed by the mother
of all *bas:* the stroke triumvirate. She had just started on a film,
Seven Women, directed by John Ford. "I don't remember anything
about the day I had the strokes, " she says. "But I was told that
after returning from the set, I was giving a bath to my daughter,
Tessa. Roald came upstairs with a martini for me and saw something was wrong. I complained about a terrible pain in my left
temple, then became disoriented, lay down on the bed, and vom-
ited." She was rushed to UCLA Medical Center, where she had
the second stroke. They immediately sent her to X-ray, and it was
discovered that a congenital aneurysm had burst in her brain.
"Then," she says, "I had the horror. The third stroke that was
supposed to do me in." But it didn't, although it did leave her
confined to a wheelchair, not able to see or speak clearly, and paralyzed on her right side. Most distressing to her was her inability
to care for her children.

She was understandably angry at her insupportable situation,
but, as she later said, "My anger stirred my resolve to get better."
She credits her then husband for the success of her post-stroke therapy. Along with relentless tough love, he devised a system of using
friends as informal therapists to keep her constantly occupied and
involved with activities that would nudge recovery forward.

"Neighbors and friends were constantly with me," she said, "walking, cooking, playing board games, to help my coordination and other activities that would force me to try speaking even the most simple words." (Dahl's program of using amateur therapists has been adopted by stroke centers around the world—thirty in England alone.) The book *Pat and Roald* by Barry Farrell describes this therapy along with other aspects of her post-stroke life.

All her help and personal hard worked paid off. Two years after her stroke, at her husband's urging, she made her first public appearance, where she delivered a speech that brought down the house—a total *haut!* After this success, the word got out and she began to receive acting offers. At first she turned them down, but again, at her husband's insistence ("God bless him!" she says), she accepted the lead in the film version of *The Subject Was Roses,* for which she received a 1968 Academy Award nomination. Rent this movie and you'll see how well her arduous therapy worked. A pen pal of ours, National Public Radio commentator Alice Furlaud, attended a dinner party where Patricia Neal was a guest. The party took place after her stroke and, Alice said, "She was remarkable, very, very normal and charming."

Also in 1968, President Johnson presented her with the "Heart of the Year" award. After this she came to realize that "I could do anything . . . with help." Since then she has appeared in numerous television productions, garnering three Emmy nominations as well as a 1971 Golden Globe Award for Best Actress in a Leading Role in a Drama Series or Television Movie for *The Homecoming.*

But the *haut* achievement that clearly means most to her was when the Fort Sanders Regional Medical Center dedicated the Patricia Neal Rehabilitation Center in Knoxville, Tennessee.

"It's a fabulous hospital," she says. "I visit several times a year, because I believe people want to see what you can come to if you work hard. Patients see that I'm not perfect. I don't walk well, can't see out of the side of my right eye . . . but I'm still up and around.

"Of course I have my little speech: 'It's so important that you work on your rehabilitation. You need people to push you for a long time . . . we now understand that recovery never ceases . . . and patients and their families can take strength in knowing that how you start out after a stroke is not the end of your life story.'"

She also imbues them with this philosophy: "A strong positive mental attitude will create more miracles than any wonder drug."

The Patricia Neal Rehabilitation Center is located in the Fort Sanders Regional Medical Center, 1901 Church Avenue, Knoxville, Tennessee 37916. For information call 1-800-Pat Neal or go to www.patneal.org.

ROBERT EVANS: FROM RAG TRADE TO RICHES

My greatest achievement is staying alive, and it ain't been easy.

—ROBERT EVANS

Long before June's stroke we had more than a casual interest in Robert Evans, producer of such blockbusters as *Love Story, Rosemary's Baby, Chinatown,* and *The Godfather.* This is because we used to wear his pants when he was a partner in the successful clothing company Evan-Picone. Then, when he was in California on a business trip relaxing by the pool at the Beverly Hills Hotel, he was discovered by Norma Shearer, who wanted him to play her late husband, Irving Thalberg, in *Man of a Thousand Faces.* After that he was tapped to be the bullfighter in *The Sun Also Rises,* over the vehement objections of everyone in the cast and crew, and even Ernest Hemingway. The head of the studio, Darryl Zanuck, overruled them all with his now immortal phrase, "The kid stays in the picture." With this, Evans realized that the power in Hollywood lies not with the actors, but with the producers. He decided he wanted to be one of those guys and so he did, rising to be head of production at Paramount. His successes and hedonistic lifestyle are chronicled in his autobiography, *The Kid Stays in the Picture* and in the documentary film by the same name, which you can—and should!—rent. At the end of the film the following epilogue appears on the screen:

> In 1998, Robert Evans suffered a severe stroke while pitching a project to Wes Craven in his screening room. Upon collapsing to the floor, Evans looked up and said, "I told you, Wes, there's never a dull moment around here."

And that's where our story begins.

"It was almost curtains for me that night," he said. He had a paralyzed left side with no feeling, and, on the way to the hospital, he was hit by another stoke. No witty remarks this time, since it deprived him of speech. But, as it turned out, if you scratched this particular hedonist, you found a stoic—albeit a reluctant one. As he put it, "Everything I love is prohibited, and everything I hate is compulsory." Any strokee will tell you the main compulsory is physical therapy—at least two hours a day and more if possible. Hate it though he did, he stuck to it and was rewarded by again being able to walk and talk and return to his old heedless lifestyle. But all play and no work has never been Evans' way. As the epilogue to the *The Kid Stays in the Picture* put it: He has since recovered and continues to produce films for Paramount Pictures. He has been at the studio for over thirty-five years. More than any other producer on the lot. Along with that he's writing a sequel to his previous memoir; this one will describe his life after stroke. He's calling it *The Fat Lady Sings,* which she almost did for Evans. We can hardly wait for it!

To show that he has a sense of humor—always an asset in stroke recovery—he allowed himself to become a cartoon character (literally) on a Comedy Central series, *Kid Notorious,* a satiric and raunchy version of his own notorious lifestyle. As long as it lasts this will no doubt increase his growing cult following. (On the Internet, it's possible to buy an "I break for Robert Evans" bumper sticker.)

His eternally youthful, upbeat attitude may have something to do with his popularity—and his recovery. "I feel that I'm only turning five this weekend," he said in a June 2002 Fox News interview. "It's been five years since my strokes. I can't believe I'm here. I shouldn't be. I died, literally. Five years ago it was like I was in cement after the strokes. Now I've put my hands in cement [in Grauman's Chinese Theater] on Hollywood Boulevard."

When he accepted the International Press Academy's 2003 Mary Pickford Award for Outstanding Artistic Contribution to the Entertainment Industry, Evans told the audience, "I'm seventy-two years old and I've stayed in the picture and so can you."

ROY HORN: THE CVA[21] OR THE TIGER? ROY'S ACCIDENT

You're probably familiar with Siegfried and Roy, "The Masters of the Impossible," and their famed act combining magic and tiger stunts if you've ever been to Las Vegas, where they've been performing for thirty years or if you've seen one of their TV specials. And if you listen to the radio or read newspapers you've undoubtedly heard of the accident of October 3, 2003, when, before a typical sold-out audience, Roy was mauled by Montecore, a 600-pound Royal White tiger and later suffered a stroke from loss of blood. Or else he suffered a stroke and the confused Montecore tried to rescue him by dragging him off stage.

[21] CVA = cerebrovascular accident (stroke)

The former theory is the one advanced by medical experts who treated him first at the University Medical Center in Las Vegas and later at UCLA. They believe that during Montecore's "mauling" a puncture wound in Roy's neck severed his vertebral artery, resulting in the massive loss of blood and the stroke that put him in a near-death situation.

The other theory, that of Siegfried, his partner of forty-six years, is that Roy lost his balance because he was having a stroke. He said that "weeks and days before the accident, Roy sometimes had high blood pressure and would say to me, 'My God! I almost passed out on stage.'"

Siegfried also dismisses reports that Montecore had been distracted by someone in the audience. He said that although a woman in the audience put up her hand, "That has happened so many times before." Siegfried believes that when Roy stumbled because of his stroke, "The cat realized Roy was not in control, so he grabbed him by the neck . . . It was not an attack, it was an accident. It was not a bite . . . and the cat was not growling. He was very gentle. Let me tell you, if it would be that the tiger would be out for killing Roy, it would have happened in no time. If he wanted to he could kill an ox in a second."

Steve Wynn, the owner of the Mirage, who hired Siegfried and Roy and who remains one of their closest friends, said that it was "a string of unfortunate events that led to the tiger carrying Roy off the stage and that it was like a tiger would carry a cub. Montecore would never attack Roy. In a way, the tiger was trying to protect him."

So there you have it—or else you don't. Was it the CVA or the tiger? If you want to learn more about the situation so you can draw your own conclusion, you can check the Internet under "Siegfried and Roy."

In the meantime we can all hope that Siegfried's enlightenment of the night of the attack turns out to be true. He was feeling lost and full of despair and "When I went to see Roy, I said to myself, 'My God, my God' . . . and then I went home and it was as if somebody gave me a hug and told me everything is going to be all right."

The doctors are cautiously optimistic but Siegfried, throwing caution to the winds, says, "I think he's going to recover everything. I have no doubt."

The most important thing, Siegfried and Roy's manager Bernie Yuman said, "is that Siegfried is really challenging him" at what will require long-term rehab. "They're enjoying these tiny triumphs."

PAMELA CRIM: THE LEGISLATIVE EYES OF TEXAS ARE ON PAMELA CRIM

Pamela Crim is by far the youngest member of our Strokee Gallery. She was only nineteen when she manifested such classic stroke symptoms as weakness in her limbs, mental confusion, one side of her face drooping, and an inability to walk or talk. The nearest hospital—a military hospital—lacked the equipment to properly diagnose Pamela's ailment, so she was taken to a neurologist sixty miles away. The neurologist considered Pamela too young to be having a stroke and thought she might just be having a really bad migraine. As good luck would have it, there was another hospital just across the street. Pamela decided to get a second opinion. There, an MRI (Magnetic Resonance Imaging) revealed that she had a massive blood clot in her brain stem, a relatively unusual stroke site. Only 10 percent of strokes occur in that area—and only around 65 percent of those who have one survive the experience. Treatment with blood thinners managed to break up the clot in Pamela's brain stem, thereby saving her life and aiding her recovery. After six months she was taken off blood thinners and prescribed an aspirin a day.

Three years later Pamela became pregnant and was put back on blood thinners. Around six weeks before her due date, her blood thinner dosage was reduced in anticipation of the delivery. Then, when she was seven months pregnant, she experienced those old familiar stroke symptoms and was given an emergency C-section. Her baby, born prematurely, had pneumonia and was flown to a children's hospital for care. The baby recovered completely.

After Pamela gave birth, the doctors again started administering tests to discover the cause of Pamela's strokes. And again they failed. Over the next two years, while living in Dallas, Pamela started experiencing repeated TIAs. Finally, in June of 2002, after months of build-up, she suffered six of these "mini-strokes" in three days.

This inspired the doctors to intensify their efforts to find the cause of Pamela's recurrent stroke problems. This time their efforts were rewarded with success. The strokes were discovered to be the result of a rare blood disease: antiphospholipid antibody. This causes the blood to regularly clot. The treatment was to take blood thinners—forever.

When Pamela was lying in the hospital after her second big stroke, she said, "I remembered a commitment I had made to God that if He healed me, I would do something big." She considered the diagnosis and successful treatment of her condition a miracle. Her husband, Lonnie, gave her that "something big" to strive for. He had heard about the Train to End Stroke Marathon Training Program put on by the American Stroke Association. Although Pamela had never in her life even run so much as a mile, train she did and was able to participate in Walt Disney World Marathon in January 2003.

But that was just the beginning. When she and her husband later moved to El Paso, Texas, Pamela ran a marathon sponsored by the El Paso American Heart Association/American Stroke

Association division. Her achievements have been recognized and lauded by the Texas Legislature with their House Resolution 958:

RESOLUTION

H.R. No. 958

WHEREAS, Pamela Crim of Allen is truly deserving of special recognition, for her determination and perseverance have served as an inspiration to all who have come to know her extraordinary story; a stroke survivor, this exceptional young woman has taken the motivation and fortitude that undergirded her recovery and applied them to helping others in the campaign against this tenacious foe; and

WHEREAS, Owing to a previously undiagnosed condition, Mrs. Crim suffered two strokes before her 25th birthday; the first, more severe, stroke occurred when she was only 19 years old; confounding her doctors' bleak predictions, she rallied and achieved a full recovery; and

WHEREAS, Several years later, when she was seven months pregnant, she suffered a second, milder stroke; she gave birth to a healthy son, however, and once again recovered fully; since then, the precipitating cause of her strokes has been determined and medication prescribed to prevent further attacks; and

WHEREAS, In the summer of 2002, Mrs. Crim learned of the American Stroke Association's Train to End Stroke Marathon Training Program, in which participants raise money for the association while preparing, with the organization's help, to run a marathon; although she had never run before, she knew immediately that this was something she wanted to do; and

WHEREAS, Persuading a coworker to serve as her "accountability partner," she joined the association's Dallas team and began training with the same focus and commitment she had brought to her earlier rehabilitation program; on January 12, 2003, she completed the Walt Disney World Marathon in Orlando, Florida—a 26.25-mile race—in 6 hours and 28 minutes; moreover, she raised $3,500 to contribute to the American Stroke Association's vital efforts; and

WHEREAS, Taking her success one step further, Mrs. Crim has signed up to participate in the marathon training program yet again; now, however, she served as a mentor for new participants as they prepared to run the Kunitake Farms Kona Marathon in Kona, Hawaii, on June 22, 2003; and

WHEREAS, Pamela Crim has not only overcome extreme life challenges, but has used them as stepping-stones to better serve others; impelled by her resilient, adventuresome spirit and her firsthand understanding of the dangers of stroke, she is making a priceless contribution to a crucial cause; now, therefore, be it

RESOLVED, That the House of Representatives of the 78th Texas Legislature hereby commend Pamela Crim on her stellar achievement in completing the Walt Disney World Marathon and on her outstanding volunteer work for the American Stroke Association and extend to her sincere best wishes for success in all of her future endeavors; and, be it further

RESOLVED, That an official copy of this resolution be prepared for Mrs. Crim as an expression of high regard by the Texas House of Representatives.

Paxton
Speaker of the House
I certify that H.R. No. 958 was adopted by the House on May 2, 2003, by a non-record vote.
Chief Clerk of the House

Ever After: Epilogue

It is difficult—perhaps impossible—to encapsulate an illness or disease, like stroke, in a book. Each stroke is different, just as each person will cope with his or her stroke differently. We do hope, however, that this book has provided a foundation for understanding stroke, recovery, and life afterwards for both strokee and caregiver, as well as being a source of comfort: You are not the only one out there battling it out.

As we all come to realize—whether strokee or caregiver—the stroke experience gives us a pungent taste of our own mortality. In the early days of her stroke and the early days of writing this book, June announced: "All I want is to live long enough to finish this book." Well, she did. So what now?

When you finish a goal, the only thing to do is create a new one. That's our plan. We're creating a Web site. Actually we're going to make it a combination Web site, where you can find information on strokes (we discover more of that every day) and a blog (which is, as www.e-blogger.com puts it, where you can freely post thoughts and interact with people). We've already reserved the Web site name: www.strokecoping.com and hope to have it up and running by the time you read this.

But until we meet again on the Internet, we want to leave you with some thoughts from Rowena Rathbone, a psychology professor friend and colleague at Los Angeles Valley College. She lived until well until her nineties, relishing every minute. In the process she formulated some secrets of success on beating old age. They included:

- **You gotta have heart.** As the song from *Damn Yankees* puts it, "When the odds are saying 'You'll never win,' that's when the grin should start." Rowena started every morning by looking in the mirror and grinning at herself.
- **You gotta have zeal.** Rowena was always excited about making plans—almost all of them including travel. She visited every continent—yes, including Antarctica—and eighty-five countries. When she died at age ninety-two, she had just returned the week before from a trip to Scotland and Paris.
- **You gotta have spunk.** At age eighty-nine, Rowena's driver's license was extended for five years. The examiner said she was the only one who passed the driving test that day. Even so, she wanted to be sure to have something to do when she could no longer drive, so she bought a computer and started taking lessons in order to enter into a whole new world at home.
- **You gotta have verve.** When she was ninety, Rowena had her car painted red.

But Rowena was just a kid compared to Jeanne Louise Clement, the oldest woman alive until she gave up her crown at one hundred twenty-two years of age. She rode her bicycle until she was one hundred and then continued walking all around her home town of Arles, France. Her advice was, "If you can't do something about it, forget about it."

And of course all that sage counsel from Rowena and Jeanne Louise is equally effective for beating strokes—if not more so. Parting words from the artist Katherine Sherwood, who suffered a stroke in her forties (her story is in "Other People's Strokes," page 201) to send you off: "Now I look at life for what it can hold, not for what it could have been."

Until we met again, so long for a while.

—*June and Barbara*

Appendix A

. . . .

How to Conquer the World with One Hand and an Attitude by Stephanie Mensh, Paul E. Berger, and Brenda Rapp, Ph.D. (Positive Power Publications, 1999)

My Year Off: Recovering Life After a Stroke by Robert McCrum (W. W. Norton, 1998)

Return to Ithaca: A Woman's Triumph Over the Disabilities of a Severe Stroke by Barbara Newborn (Element Books, 1997)

After Stroke by David M. Hinds and Peter Morris (Thorsons Publishers, 2000)

Slow Dance: A Story of Stroke, Love, and Disability by Bonnie Sherr Klein (Page Mill Press, 1998)

The Diving Bell and the Butterfly: A Memoir of Life in Death by Jean-Dominique Bauby and Jeremy Leggett (Knopf, 1997)

My Stroke of Luck by Kirk Douglas (William Morrow, 2002)

After the Stroke by May Sarton (W. W. Norton, 1990)

Cyclops Awakes: A Newspaperman Fights Back After a Massive Stroke by John E. Mantle (Lucky Press, 2000)

Stroke of Luck: Life, Crisis, and Rebirth of a Stroke Survivor by Howard Rocket with Rachel Sklar (Parnassus, 1999)

Appendix B

STROKE ORGANIZATIONS

. . . .

American Stroke Association:
   A Division of American Heart Association
7272 Greenville Avenue
Dallas, TX 75231-4596
strokeassociation@heart.org
www.strokeassociation.org
Tel: 1-888-4STROKE (478-7653)
Fax: 214-706-5231

Brain Aneurysm Foundation
12 Clarendon Street
Boston, MA 02116
information@bafound.org
www.bafound.org
Tel: 617-723-3870
Fax: 617-723-8672

National Stroke Association
9707 East Easter Lane
Englewood, CO 80112-3747
info@stroke.org
www.stroke.org
Tel: 303-649-9299; 800-STROKES (787-6537)
Fax: 303-649-1328

Stroke Clubs International
805 12th Street
Galveston, TX 77550
strokeclubs@earthlink.net
Tel: 409-762-1022

National Aphasia Association
29 John Street
Suite 1103
New York, NY 10038
naa@aphasia.org
www.aphasia.org
Tel: 212-267-2814; 800-922-4NAA (4622)
Fax: 212-267-2812

Children's Hemiplegia and Stroke Assocn. (CHASA)
4101 West Green Oaks Blvd.
PMB #149
Arlington, TX 76016
info5@chasa.org
www.hemikids.org
Tel: 817-492-4325

Hazel K. Goddess Fund for Stroke Research in Women
785 Park Avenue
New York, NY 10021-3552
courtneymartin@thegoddessfund.org
www.thegoddessfund.org
Tel: 212-734-8067
Fax: 212-288-2160

American Health Assistance Foundation
22512 Gateway Center Drive
Clarksburg, M.D. 20871
info@ahaf.org
www.ahaf.org
Tel: 301-948-3244; 800-437-AHAF (2423)
Fax: 301-258-9454

Index

weight gain and control, caregiver, 124,
164–69
wheelchairs, 20, 82–83
word games to restore brain function,
137–38

xylitol gum, 51

yoga, 171–73

Zanaflex, 45
Zen meditation, 161,
163–64
Zen philosophy, 95–99
Zocor (simvastatin), 61